Musculoskeletal Disease and Obesity

John M. O´Byrne • Fiachra Rowan
Alan Molloy
Editors

Musculoskeletal Disease and Obesity

Multi-disciplinary Interventions

Springer

Editors
John M. O´Byrne
RCSI University of Medicine and Health Sciences
Department of Orthopaedic Surgery
National Orthopaedic Hospital
Cappagh, Dublin, Ireland

Fiachra Rowan
Dept. of Orthopaedic Surgery
University Hospital Waterford
Waterford, Ireland

Alan Molloy
Dept. of Orthopaedic Surgery
National Orthopaedic Hospital, Cappagh
Dublin, Ireland

ISBN 978-3-031-63309-6 ISBN 978-3-031-63310-2 (eBook)
https://doi.org/10.1007/978-3-031-63310-2

This Springer imprint is published by the registered company Springer Nature Switzerland AG
The registered company address is: Gewerbestrasse 11, 6330 Cham, Switzerland

To my wife, Dr. Fiona Kearns, who has filled my life with joy.

—John M. O'Byrne

To my wife Claire and my children Oscar, Quinn, Molly, and Teddy: these are the days!

—Fiachra Rowan

To my wife Leann and my children Eve and Rebecca. Thank you for everything.

—Alan Molloy

Foreword

With obesity reaching epidemic proportions in many developed countries, there are significant implications on how we approach the surgical treatment of orthopaedic patients. Obesity is an independent risk factor for the development of osteoarthritis. As its prevalence rises so does the need for joint replacements and orthopaedic interventions in obese patients.

A significant issue is that the obese patient population provides unique challenges for successful surgical treatment. Physically, due to the patient's size and body habitus, the surgical approach and exposure, positioning of the patient, and execution of the procedure are significantly more challenging compared to non-obese patients. These physical challenges mandate the use of more resources in their care. Medically, obese patients have more comorbidities, putting them at risk for adverse surgical outcomes. These comorbidities, including sleep apnea diabetes, and cardiovascular issues require higher levels of care and preoperative evaluation. While there is no clear consensus, some studies have shown that these patients may be subject to higher rates of complications and poor outcomes.

A thorough understanding of the challenges in execution and management of surgery in the obese is required for successful outcomes. It is not adequate to simply repeat the usual steps performed in the average patient. The authors present a thoughtful consideration of the technical aspects necessary for successful management of obese patients and how to overcome the challenges inherent in their care. This book gives a complete review on orthopaedic subspecialty and a review of implications for anaesthesia and rehabilitation issues. For clinicians caring for the obese, this book provides an essential strategic outline for success.

Hospital for Special Surgery
New York, NY, USA

Michael L. Parks

Preface

As editors, we are delighted to present this textbook outlining the range of musculoskeletal challenges in patients living with obesity.

The epidemic of obesity is well described and increasingly realised to be a challenge for healthcare professionals and healthcare providers. The early chapters in this textbook look at the epidemiology and pathogenesis and also examine medical and surgical treatments. The musculoskeletal chapters focus on the different parts of the body where obesity contributes to the pathology and complicates the management. Specific chapters focus on paediatrics, oncology, and sports injuries. Imaging of patients living with obesity and also anaesthetic issues arising in this group of patients are highlighted. Rehabilitation of patients living with obesity is also described.

Obesity continues to challenge patients, clinicians, and providers, and we hope this textbook will prove a useful guide to anyone involved in the care of musculoskeletal conditions that arise in this patient population.

We thank all the chapter authors, and we particularly acknowledge the invaluable support of Ms. Ursula Gormally in the preparation of this textbook.

Dublin, Ireland — John M. O'Byrne
Dublin, Ireland — Alan Molloy
Waterford, Ireland — Fiachra Rowan
June 2024

Contents

Contributors

Ryan Alexander, MSc, CAT Dublin City University, UPMC Sports Surgery Clinic, Dublin, Ireland

Aoife Brady, MB, BCh, BAO, MCAI Beaumont Hospital, Dublin, Ireland

University Hospital Waterford, Dublin, Ireland

Laura Browne, MB, BCh, BAO St James's Hospital, Dublin, Ireland

Adrian Cassar-Gheiti, MD, FRCSI, FRCS (Tr&Orth) National Orthopaedic Hospital Cappagh, Dublin, Ireland

John T. Cassidy, MCh, FRCS (Tr&Orth) Croom Orthopaedic Hospital/ University Hospital Limerick, Limerick, Ireland

Stacey Darwish, MB, ChB, FRCS (Ed) T&O National Spine Injuries Unit, Mater Misericordiae University Hospital and National Orthopaedic Hospital Cappagh, Dublin, Ireland

Brian M. Devitt, MD, MMedSci, PhD, FRCS Dublin City University, UPMC Sports Surgery Clinic, Dublin, Ireland

Patrick Devitt, MB, BCh, BAO Mater Misericordiae University Hospital, Dublin, Ireland

Colin Dunlevy, PhD, MISCP Centre for Obesity Management, St. Columcille's Hospital, Dublin, Ireland

Ciara M. Egan, MB, MCh, MRCS, FRCS Children's Health Ireland at Crumlin Children's Hospital, Dublin, Ireland

Sarah K. Eustace, MB, BCh, BAO National Orthopaedic Hospital Cappagh, Dublin, Ireland

Stephen J. Eustace Newman Professor of Radiology-University College Dublin, Dublin, Ireland

CNOH and MMUH and Mater Private Hospitals, Dublin, Ireland

National Orthopaedic Hospital Cappagh, Dublin, Ireland

Alan Gaffney, MB, BCh, PhD Beaumont Hospital, Dublin, Ireland

Orna Alexandra Glynn, MB, BCh, BAO National Orthopaedic Hospital Cappagh, Dublin, Ireland

Michael Hanlon, MB, BCh, BAO National Orthopaedic Hospital Cappagh, Dublin, Ireland

Helen Heneghan, MB, BCh, BAO, PhD, FRCS St. Vincent's University Hospital, Dublin, Ireland

Olivia Horner, MB, BCh, BAO Tallaght University Hospital, Dublin, Ireland

Allison Kelliher, MB, BCh, BAO Royal College of Surgeons in Ireland, Dublin, Ireland

National Orthopaedic Hospital Cappagh, Dublin, Ireland

Andrew Kelly, MB, BCh, BAO National Spine Injuries Unit, NCHD, Mater Misericordiae University Hospital, Dublin, Ireland

UCD School of Medicine, Dublin, Ireland

Orlaith Kelly, MB, BCh, BAO, PDip, MRCSI Royal College of Surgeons Ireland, RCSI, Dublin, Ireland

Ailbhe Kenny, MB, BCh, BAO St. James's Hospital, Dublin, Ireland

National Orthopaedic Hospital Cappagh, Dublin, Ireland

Fred Kenny, MISCP, MB, BCh, BAO National Orthopaedic Hospital Cappagh, Dublin, Ireland

Eisten Tillie Keogh, BA Mod. School of Medicine, Royal College of Surgeons in Ireland, Dublin, Ireland

Lyndon Y. H. Low, MB, BCh, BAO, MCh, MRCSI University College Hospital, Galway, Ireland

Royal College of Surgeons Ireland, Dublin 2, Ireland

Rosanne-Sara Lynham, MB, BAO, BCh, MA(Hon), MCh, MRCS Dublin City University, UPMC Sports Surgery Clinic, Dublin, Ireland

National Orthopaedic Hospital Cappagh, Dublin, Ireland

Matthew Macciacchera, BMSc, MB, BCh, BAO Royal College of Surgeons in Ireland, Dublin, Ireland

Nuala McAuley, MRCSI National Orthopaedic Hospital Cappagh, Dublin, Ireland

Royal College of Surgeons Ireland, Dublin 2, Ireland

Stephen McLoughlin Royal College of Surgeons in Ireland, Dublin, Ireland

University of Limerick, Limerick City, Ireland

Conor McNamee National Spine Injuries Unit, Mater Misericordiae University Hospital, Dublin, Ireland

UCD School of Medicine, Dublin, Ireland

Adeel Memon, MBBS, MCh, FRCS (Tr&Orth) Mater Private Hospital, Dublin, Ireland

Mater Private Network Cork, Cork, Ireland

Peggy Miller, MB, BCh, BAO, MCh National Orthopaedic Hospital Cappagh, Dublin, Ireland

University Hospital Waterford, Waterford, Ireland

Royal College of Surgeons Ireland, Dublin 2, Ireland

Alan P. Molloy, FRCS (Tr&Orth) University College Dublin, Dublin, Ireland

St. Vincent's University and National Orthopaedic Cappagh Hospitals, Dublin, Ireland

Barry Moran, MB, BCh, BAO, MRCPI St. Vincent's University Hospital, Dublin, Ireland

Colin Murphy, MCh, FEBOT, FRCS (Tr&Orth) Galway University Hospitals, Galway, Ireland

Aisling O'Byrne, MB, BCh, BAO Trinity College Dublin, TCD, Dublin, Ireland

Barry O'Neill, MB, MCh, MRCSI, FRCS Sligo Regional University Hospital, Sligo, Ireland

Donal O'Shea, MB, BCh, BAO, MD, FRCPI, FRCP St. Vincent's University Hospital, Loughlinstown Hospital, University College, Dublin, Ireland

Gary C. O'Toole, FRCS (Tr&Orth) St. Vincent's and National Orthopaedic Hospital Cappagh, Dublin, Ireland

Brian Quinn, BSc, MB, BCh, BAO Department of Nephrology, Cork University Hospital, Cork City, Ireland

Ailbhe Rogan Dublin City University, Dublin, Ireland

Bisola Salaja, MB, BCh, BAO, MRCS University College Hospital/Merlin Park Regional Hospital, Galway, Ireland

National Orthopaedic Hospital Cappagh, Dublin, Ireland

John Scanlon, MCh, BCh Royal College of Surgeons in Ireland, Dublin, Ireland

Hugo C. Temperley, MB, BCh, BAO Department of Surgery, Trinity Centre for Health Sciences, St. James's Hospital and Trinity College Dublin, Dublin, Ireland

NCHD, Dublin, Ireland

Alexander Vincent, BM, BCh, BAO, MSc Royal College of Surgeons in Ireland, Dublin 2, Ireland

Pathogenesis, Prevalence and Epidemiology of Obesity

1

Brian Quinn, Laura Browne, and Donal O'Shea

1.1 Introduction

Obesity is defined by the World Health Organization (WHO) as an excessive accumulation of body fat which presents a risk to health [1]. The WHO recommend measuring a person's body fat content using the body mass index (BMI) calculation [1, 2]. The different classifications of weight are shown in Table 1.1.

$$\mathrm{BMI} = \frac{\mathrm{Weight}\,(\mathrm{in\ kg})}{(\mathrm{Height\ in\ Metres})^2}$$

Table 1.1 WHO BMI ranges and classifications [1]

WHO classification	BMI range
Underweight	<18.4
Normal	18.5–24.9
Overweight	25–29.9
Obese	>30

B. Quinn (✉)
Department of Nephrology, Cork University Hospital, Cork City, Republic of Ireland
e-mail: 118703741@umail.ucc.ie

L. Browne
St James's Hospital, Dublin, Ireland
e-mail: Brownel4@tcd.ie

D. O'Shea
St. Vincent's University Hospital, Loughlinstown Hospital, University College, Dublin, Ireland
e-mail: info@dosheaendo.ie

J. M. O´Byrne et al. (eds.), *Musculoskeletal Disease and Obesity*,
https://doi.org/10.1007/978-3-031-63310-2_1

Although BMI is the gold standard used for assessing obesity, it has several flaws with its implementation. BMI measures body mass but does not distinguish between lean body mass and fat body mass. Therefore, using BMI to measure an athlete or bodybuilder would lead that individual to be classified as clinically obese. Additionally, the ranges specified by the WHO for BMI do not adequately account for height variability that occurs between phenotypes. This means that BMI can be properly employed as a measuring tool in America and Europe [3–6] while it fails to adequately assess obesity prevalence in Asia [1, 2]. A proposed remedy for this is to lower the cutoff ranges of overweight and obese BMI limits so that they reflect the country's average height ranges [7].

Alternative methods of measuring body fat are body fat percentage, which more accurately assesses fat content, and hip:waist ratio. However, these measurements are not broadly employed to assess a person's body fat content [2].

1.2 Incidence and Prevalence of Obesity in the Modern Day

Obesity has been recognised as a risk to health since the nineteenth century [1], and yet the prevalence of obesity has gradually increased over the past 100 years. As of 2016, almost 2 billion people were found to be overweight worldwide [14]. Current projections have the global population reaching 1 billion obese adults by 2025 [14]. The continents with the highest obese population are shown in Table 1.2.

As the prevalence of obesity rises globally, so does its disease burden. Obesity has been recognised as a pro-inflammatory condition which can in turn promote the development of musculoskeletal disease, type 2 diabetes and specific cancers [1–4]. Furthermore, it is a significant contributor to cardiovascular disease and respiratory disorders. Additionally, a frequently overlooked aspect of obesity is the effect it has on an individual's mental health. As of 2014 the economic burden of obesity was estimated at US$2 trillion globally [17]. This figure was generated based on the number of days missed due to sick leave, combined with the cost of medical interventions for individuals in which obesity was a contributing factor to their illness.

Table 1.2 Prevalence of obesity globally as of 2015 [7]

	Geographical location	Overweight prevalence as of 2015 (%)	Obese prevalence as of 2015 (%)
1	Americas	64.2	28.3
2	Europe	59.6	22.9
3	East Mediterranean	49.6	19.6
4	Africa	34	12.7
5	West Pacific	28.2	4.9
6	Southeast Asia	22	5

1.3 Pathogenesis

The metabolic pathway for the generation of fat is called lipogenesis. It begins in the brain, where hormones regulating starvation/satiety levels in the body will dictate whether the body is hungry or not. The individual will feel hungry and eat [7, 8]. Food is then metabolised. The process by which the body will turn ingested nutrients into energy is called the Krebs cycle [8]. This will lead to the generation of energy from the breakdown of glucose.

When there is an excess of glucose, the body will then attempt to store it in the form of fat. It is the body's attempt to create stores of energy that can be utilised in times of need [8]. Glucose is converted to fatty acids which are then turned into triglycerides. This occurs in the liver and fat cells (adipocytes).

Lipogenesis has a counterpart called lipolysis. It is the dissolution of lipids to generate energy. This is how the body will access its stores of energy.

The balance between lipogenesis and lipolysis is a dynamic one. In times of abundant food access and low-energy demand, lipogenesis will prevail over lipolysis. The opposite is also true.

1.4 Factors Contributing to Obesity

1.4.1 Diet

Typically, high-calorie diets will accelerate lipogenesis and thus increase the prevalence of obesity [7–12]. Foods such as unprocessed red meats, processed meats, sugar-sweetened foods and foods with high levels of saturated fats, trans fats, dietary cholesterol and sodium have been linked with higher rates of obesity [9–12]. Similarly, foods that will reduce rates of obesity are fruits, vegetables, beans, legumes, nuts, seeds, wholegrain, milk, polyunsaturated fats, fish and food containing omega-3 and high-content dietary fibre [9–12].

Diet is highly dependent on geographical factors [9–11]. Typically, a country will eat what it can make. Countries living by the sea will have selections of seafood while in landlocked countries, seafood is more difficult to come by and therefore more expensive. Diet is also dependent on a country's socio-economic status. A rich country that cannot grow exotic fruits can import them for a high price. Conversely, a developing country will have to rely on seasonal fruits and vegetables rather than importing fruits and vegetables all year round.

A factor common to all countries is that the availability of cheap but nutrient-poor food is becoming more and more abundant [9, 10]. Processed food with long shelf lives can be made, transported and stored with relatively low cost and difficulty. The same cannot be said for fresh ingredients such as fruit. This leads there to be an ease of access to nutrient-poor, lipogenic foodstuffs [9, 10].

So, to briefly summarise, a person's diet is limited to the food that is available in that country and is further limited to what that person can afford. This means that a wealthy individual in a wealthy country will have a wide variety of food to choose from and conversely, a poor individual in a poor country will be limited to the cheaper foodstuffs available in that country [9].

Surprisingly, countries with the highest degree of food availability also have the highest rates of obesity [5]. Continents such as the Americas and Europe have the highest prevalence of obesity and contain the wealthiest countries in the world [7]. In general, rich countries will have a higher degree of obesity than poorer countries [3, 7, 11]. However, the rate of change of obesity prevalence within those countries is different [7, 11]. Rich countries are generally seeing a decline in the rate of change of obesity prevalence [7, 11]. This means that, although people are still gaining weight, there are less of them with each passing year. Conversely, in developing countries the rate of change is increasing. Some of the factors contributing to this phenomenon are access to healthcare, food education and access to better foodstuffs [7, 9].

1.4.2 Genetics

A person's genetic makeup has a variety of effects on their growth and development. Weight gain is influenced by monogenic mutations and polygenic mutations [13–16]. Monogenic mutations are single genes that differ from the standard version of the gene. Their mutation leads to their expression patterns being different to what would be considered normal. The role of these genes is so impactful that they can drastically alter an individual's phenotype [15]. Examples of monogenic mutations are as follows: leptin (LEP), leptin receptor (LEPR), proopiomelanocortin (POMC) and melanocortin 4 receptor (MC4R) [13, 14]. Possessing any one of these mutations has been directly linked to excessive lipogenesis [13, 14]. These genetic mutations are rare and usually associated with developmental disabilities such as Prader–Willi syndrome [13]. Individuals with these genetic mutations will present as obese in early life, around late childhood or adolescence [13]. These genes display a high degree of heritability, meaning that an individual with these mutations has a 40–70% chance of passing the mutations on to their offspring [15].

Polygenic genes are multiple mutations that will collectively contribute to an increase in lipogenesis [15]. They are more commonly seen and can include hundreds of single-nucleotide polymorphisms (SNPs) [15]. Compared to monogenic mutations, these polygenic mutations will have a modest effect on lipogenesis [15]. Furthermore, they have a significantly lower heritability compared to their monogenic counterparts [15]. There is evidence showing that polygenic mutations are strongly linked to environmental factors [15]. A direct comparison between the two types of influential genes is presented in Fig. 1.1.

Monogenic	Polygenic
• Early Onset disease (paediatric)	• Late onset disease
• Single gene mutation has huge impact	• Hundreds of genetic mutations have small impact
• High genetic burden/penetrance	• Low genetic burden/penetrance
• Only a handful of genes	• Hundreds of variants
• Influenced by inheritance	• Influenced by environment
• Rare	• Common

Fig. 1.1 Comparison between monogenic vs. polygenic mutations [15]

1.4.3 Current Disease Modelling

Previous disease modelling on obesity was a simple input/output model [12]. An individual will ingest a specific number of calories a day. The individual will utilise a certain amount of those calories as energy throughout the day. The remainder of the calories are stored or excreted. This model assumed a linear correlation between energy input and output. However, more recent research has shown the correlation to be more dynamic and that it is influenced by factors such as basal metabolic rate, thermic effect of feeding and physical activity [12].

This could explain why obese individuals find it so difficult to continuously lose weight with diet and exercise. When an obese individual is put on a diet and exercise regimen, they will begin to lose weight quickly then stabilise and lose a lower but continuous amount of weight [12].

One of the models currently used for weight gain/weight loss is the constrained model of energy expenditure. This model states that the body will utilise a fixed constant amount of energy within a day. This energy will be split between active and passive processes. When more active energy is required, passive processes are altered to change the energy balance in favour of active processes [12].

1.5 Overview and Summary

To recap this chapter:

- Body mass is assessed using the body mass index equation.
- Obesity is the excessive accumulation of fat tissue that presents a risk to health.
- The generation of fat tissue is called lipogenesis.

- The factors influencing the rate of lipogenesis include diet, genetics, geographical location and socio-economic factors.
- Obesity was once thought of as a simple in/out process but has since been recognised as a dynamic multifactorial process.

References

1. Berghöfer A, Pischon T, Reinhold T, et al. Obesity prevalence from a European perspective: a systematic review. BMC Public Health. 2008;8:200.
2. Marques A, Peralta M, Naia A, Loureiro N, de Matos MG. Prevalence of adult overweight and obesity in 20 European countries, 2014. Eur J Pub Health. 2018;28(2):295–300.
3. Ogden CL, Carroll MD, Fryar CD, Flegal KM. Prevalence of obesity among adults and youth: United States, 2011–2014. NCHS Data Brief. 2015;219:1–8.
4. Hales CM, Carroll MD, Fryar CD, Ogden CL. Prevalence of obesity among adults and youth: United States, 2015–2016. NCHS Data Brief. 2017;288:1–8.
5. Janssen F, Bardoutsos A, Vidra N. Obesity prevalence in the long-term future in 18 European countries and in the USA. Obes Facts. 2020;13:514–27.
6. Buoncristiano M, Spinelli A, Williams J, Nardone P, Rito AI, García-Solano M, Grøholt EK, Gutiérrez-González E, Klepp KI, Starc G, Petrauskienė A. Childhood overweight and obesity in Europe: changes from 2007 to 2017. Obes Rev. 2021;22:e13226.
7. Chooi YC, Ding C, Magkos F. The epidemiology of obesity. Metabolism. 2019;92:6–10.
8. Kersten S. Mechanisms of nutritional and hormonal regulation of lipogenesis. EMBO Rep. 2001;2(4):282–6.
9. La Vecchia C, Majem LS. Evaluating trends in global dietary patterns. Lancet Glob Health. 2015;3(3):e114–5.
10. Popkin BM, Hawkes C. Sweetening of the global diet, particularly beverages: patterns, trends, and policy responses. Lancet Diabetes Endocrinol. 2016;4(2):174–86.
11. Imamura F, Micha R, Khatibzadeh S, Fahimi S, Shi P, Powles J, Mozaffarian D. Dietary quality among men and women in 187 countries in 1990 and 2010: a systematic assessment. Lancet Glob Health. 2015;3(3):e132–42.
12. Pontzer H. Constrained total energy expenditure and the evolutionary biology of energy balance. Exerc Sport Sci Rev. 2015;43(3):110–6.
13. Nguyen DM, El-Serag HB. The epidemiology of obesity. Gastroenterol Clin. 2010;39(1):1–7.
14. Yang W, Kelly T, He J. Genetic epidemiology of obesity. Epidemiol Rev. 2007;29(1):49–61.
15. Loos RJ, Yeo GS. The genetics of obesity: from discovery to biology. Nat Rev Genet. 2022;23(2):120–33.
16. Herrera BM, Lindgren CM. The genetics of obesity. Curr Diab Rep. 2010;10:498–505.
17. Tremmel M, Gerdtham UG, Nilsson PM, Saha S. Economic burden of obesity: a systematic literature review. Int J Environ Res Public Health. 2017;14(4):435.

2 Medical Treatment of Obesity

Patrick Devitt, Barry Moran, and Donal O'Shea

2.1 Introduction

Obesity is a major health problem leading to significant morbidity and mortality in the modern world. Obesity is defined by the WHO as an 'abnormal or excessive fat accumulation that presents a risk to health' and is classified by the body mass index (BMI), the parameters of which are shown below [1].

Overweight: BMI 25–29.9 kg/m^2
Obese (class I): BMI ≥30 kg/m^2–<35 kg/m^2
Obese (class II): BMI ≥35 kg/m^2 and <40 kg/m^2
Obese (class III) ≥40 kg/m^2

The WHO considers the issue an 'epidemic' and estimates an annual death toll of over 4 million people dying as a result of the complications of being overweight or obese. The rates of obesity have risen dramatically in recent decades. Between 2000 and 2010, there was an increase in the population with a BMI > 30 kg/m^2 of approximately 40%, an increase of >80% of people with a BMI > 40 kg/m^2, and an increase of 120% in those with a BMI > 50 [2]. This demonstrates an asymmetric relative increase in those suffering from class III obesity. It correlates with

P. Devitt (✉)
Mater Misericordiae University Hospital, Dublin, Ireland
e-mail: devittp1@tcd.ie

B. Moran
St. Vincent's University Hospital, Dublin, Ireland

D. O'Shea
St. Vincent's University Hospital, Loughlinstown Hospital, University College, Dublin, Ireland
e-mail: info@dosheaendo.ie

J. M. O´Byrne et al. (eds.), *Musculoskeletal Disease and Obesity*,
https://doi.org/10.1007/978-3-031-63310-2_2

numerous health consequences, including cardiovascular disease and stroke, which are the leading causes of death worldwide. It is also associated with diabetes, hypertension, obstructive sleep apnoea, osteoarthritis, and certain cancers, including endometrial, breast, ovarian, prostate, liver, gallbladder, and colon cancers [3]. Higher BMI has also been correlated with an increase in mortality, which has been established in systematic reviews [4, 5]. Systematic reviews and meta-analyses confirm that weight loss is effective at reducing complications and morbidity associated with obesity but a direct mortality benefit resulting from weight loss has not yet been established [6]. The importance of weight reduction is rooted in mitigating these complications. In this chapter, we will take a look at the full picture when deciding to institute medical treatment for obesity and its associated complications—looking at both conservative and lifestyle-based therapies, pharmacotherapies, and when to consider referral for surgical intervention. Obesity is a complicated condition, and despite mainstream beliefs, sedentary lifestyle and increased caloric intake are not the sole causes of obesity. It is a complex mix of genetic and environmental factors that, when combined, create the conditions for weight gain. The clinician should adopt a holistic treatment strategy best fitting for the individual patient at hand.

2.2 Evaluation and Risk Assessment

The first step when deciding to institute a management plan is prompt recognition of the condition, determination of a cause, and a risk assessment. The clinician should identify the patient as being overweight or obese, accurately assess BMI, and document this clearly in the medical record. The 2013 AHA/ACC/TOS guidelines also suggest measuring waist circumference in patients with BMI 25–34.9 kg/m^2 as it provides additional information on cardiometabolic risk [7]. Waist circumference is an independent risk factor for cardiovascular disease, dyslipidaemia, and non-alcoholic fatty liver disease and it is considered a component of the 'metabolic syndrome'. A waist circumference measurement is not necessary if the patient's BMI is >35 kg/m^2 as it is likely to be elevated anyway and will not lend any further information. A further risk assessment should take place with screening for additional cardiovascular risk factors and complications of obesity. A thorough history and physical examination should be undertaken, including measuring of blood pressure, and laboratory tests looking at thyroid function tests, fasting glucose or glycated haemoglobin, liver function tests, and a lipid profile. The clinician should consider and rule out secondary causes as clinically indicated, including endocrine disease (thyroid disease/Cushing disease/polycystic ovarian syndrome) and medication-induced weight gain. Common medications leading to weight gain include anti-hypoglycaemic agents such as sulfonylureas, thiazolidinediones, glucocorticoids, antipsychotics, and antidepressants. The recent cessation of smoking can also contribute. This is an important point to note as in many circumstances the benefit of smoking cessation outweighs the risks of weight gain. The history of weight gain, including previous weight loss attempts, lifestyle, dietary, and family history, can also be useful and can tailor individual weight loss plans and targets for the patient. If established cardiovascular disease, cardiovascular risk factors, or complications of obesity such as sleep apnoea, type 2 diabetes, etc., have developed at this point, then the patient is deemed very high risk.

Once these risk factors are established, the next step is to identify the candidates who are deemed suitable for weight loss interventions. The aims of treatment are to prevent/mitigate the complications of weight gain and improve the patient's quality of life. Because of the correlation of health risks and mortality associated with an increase in BMI, any patient with a BMI of >25 kg/m^2 is an appropriate candidate for weight loss interventions but evidence is sparse on specific BMI targets. Those with a BMI between 25 and 29.9 kg/m^2 without further risk factors should be counselled in the primary care setting about the risks of further weight gain and on conservative weight loss interventions, including diet, exercise, and monitoring of their weight.

Minimal risk includes patients with a BMI of 20–25 kg/m^2 unless there is an elevated waist circumference. Asian individuals have an increased cardiometabolic risk even at lower BMIs, so it is especially important that a weight circumference be measured in this population even if not deemed overweight by the WHO classification [8].

Low-risk candidates include those with a BMI of 25–29 kg/m^2 who do not have cardiovascular disease risk factors or other complications related to excess weight. These individuals receive counselling and dietary/exercise advice.

Moderate-risk candidates include those with a BMI of 30–24.9 kg/m^2 without other complicating comorbidities. Those with a BMI of 25–29.9 but with a complication of obesity/further risk factors also fall into this category. These individuals should receive an intensive, multidisciplined approach to weight loss management [9].

High-risk individuals are those with a BMI of >35 kg/m^2, and in those with a BMI > 30 with established complications and risk factors. These individuals should receive the most aggressive form of weight-lowering therapy [10].

2.3 Management Strategies

The management of obesity has evolved in recent years; however, it remains focused on three core strategies: comprehensive lifestyle intervention (including diet, exercise behaviour modification, psychotherapy), pharmacotherapy, and surgical intervention. It is a complex and individualised process. The clinician must consider both the urgency of weight loss and the realistic targets that can be met. The motivation and personal goals of the patient are also important in implanting a successful strategy. The decision to implement weight loss measures should be weighed against competing priorities. For example, if a patient is smoking or has recently suffered an acute MI, then smoking cessation, risk factor optimisation, and cardiac rehabilitation take priority, with weight loss being a secondary goal. Generally, a weight loss target of 5–7% of total body weight generates significant health and benefits to quality of life. This target is generally achievable within 6 months for most patients, especially those who have not sought formal weight loss interventions before. High-risk individuals or moderate-risk individuals failing conservative therapy should receive referral to specialists. Ideally patients should be managed as part of a multidisciplinary team, including physicians, bariatric surgeons, dietitians, psychotherapists, and nurse practitioners.

2.3.1 Conservative Strategies

Dietitians are preferably consulted for counselling on dietary plans. The main component of a dietary strategy is simply reducing overall caloric intake [11]. Interestingly, however, meta-analyses do not show a difference in long-term weight loss for very-low-calorie diets (<800 kcal per day) [12]. However, short-term weight loss can be achieved, and this method of dietary restriction can be useful if requiring rapid weight loss, for example, preoperatively. Exercise programs are generally not as effective as dietary restriction but are an important adjunct. They also improve cardiovascular health [13].

Behavioural modification helps make changes in the patient's eating behaviour and is conducted by psychologists/dietitians and other trained professionals. The 2013 guidelines suggest an intensive, multidisciplinary, in-person comprehensive strategy focusing on those three core principles by trained interventionalists with at least 14 in-person sessions over 6 months. To prevent regain of weight, they recommend participation in maintenance programs with at least monthly counselling for a further year [7]. However, it is clear in practice that this is an unrealistic expectation for the majority of patients, so would be reserved for the most severe cases. Unfortunately, longer term outcomes of conservative management have not been successful in maintaining weight loss [14]. These are possibly due to a complex mix of hormonal and metabolic adaptations that promote weight gain after initial successful weight loss. However, even if conservative methods do not meet the desired outcomes, the management team should continue optimisation of diet/exercise and behavioural modification alongside more intensive therapy.

2.3.2 Pharmacotherapy

Failing conservative measures, the decision then becomes whether to institute pharmacological or surgical therapy in addition to lifestyle modifications. It is also at this point that the primary care clinician should consider referral to a specialist obesity clinic. The clinician should also carefully balance the potential side effects of any intervention against the benefits. In the setting of weight-related comorbidities, it is important to avoid medications that may exacerbate weight gain. For example, in the obese patient with type 2 diabetes, anti-hypoglycaemic agents can promote the gaining or loss of weight, or can be weight neutral [15] The clinician should, in the absence of other contraindications, generally try and tailor the treatment of comorbid conditions to account for their weight status.

Guidelines suggest that appropriate candidates for drug therapy include patients with

BMI ≥ 30 kg/m^2
Or
BMI of 27–29 kg/m^2 with weight-related complications or comorbidities

Those who would meet the criteria for treatment ideally should have failed to meet a weight loss target of ≥5% of total body weight with lifestyle interventions [16]. Options include glucagon-like peptide receptor analogues (semaglutide or liraglutide), the combination drug phentermine-extended release topiramate, combination bupropion–naltrexone, orlistat, sympathomimetic drugs such as phentermine, diethylpropion, and phendimetrazine. Meta-analyses do confirm the efficacy of weight loss with these medications when compared to placebo; however, there is a lack of reporting of side effects and length of action, as well as a lack of head-to-head comparisons [17–19]. Monitoring of patients on all medical therapy should include weight, blood pressure, and heart rate every 4–6 weeks. Blood sugar levels should be monitored in diabetics as weight loss can precipitate hypoglycaemic episodes. The clinician should also regularly assess the patient's mood and be vigilant for psychiatric symptoms as several of these medications can have neuropsychiatric side effects. Generally, if a patient does not lose 4–5% body weight after 12 weeks of therapy at the maximal tolerated dose, then the drug is discontinued and another agent can then be trialled.

2.3.2.1 GLP-1 Agonists

GLP-1 agonists have changed modern practice in terms of obesity management. While evidence of their benefits to weight loss is incontrovertible, they generate significant controversy mostly due to their cost and have a side effect profile that must be taken into account. Off-license demand for them has soared, and they have generated significant media interest due to restrictions to their access and celebrity endorsement. First used for the treatment of type 2 diabetes, they were also found to have a weight loss effect, which led to their study in the treatment of obesity. There is strong evidence from several RCTs showing their effectiveness for obesity management both in diabetics and non-diabetics. They are now the first line even for non-diabetics in the absence of contraindications or intolerance.

The two GLP-1 agonists liraglutide and semaglutide are the mainstays of this class used for obesity treatment. They are available as once-daily or once-weekly subcutaneous injections, respectively. They stimulate glucose-dependent insulin secretion and inhibit gastric emptying, leading to slower digestion of food and increased satiety. They can also inhibit the feeding centre in the CNS, thus reducing appetite [20]. It is also possible that their side effects of nausea and vomiting are a contributing factor to the weight loss effect seen. Their advantage is the concurrent treatment of type 2 diabetes mellitus in comorbid obese patients; however, as stated, they are not limited to this cohort [21, 22].

Liraglutide was the first medication of the class of GLP-1 agonists to be approved by the US FDA for the management of obesity. The disadvantage of it compared to semaglutide is it is a once-daily injectable administration compared to once-weekly for semaglutide. Limiting factors for both of these agents are gastrointestinal side effects such as nausea and vomiting, as well as the adverse effects of pancreatitis, gallstones, and renal impairment (although these are much rarer). Symptoms of these should be monitored closely. Clinically, it is used at higher doses to achieve its weight reduction benefits (3 mg/day) [23]. A randomised, double-blind, placebo-controlled study involving over 550 patients at different liraglutide doses, placebo, and orlistat with a BMI between 30 and 40 kg/m^2 had an average weight loss of 4.8–7.2 kg at doses of 1.2 mg/day, 1.8 mg/day, 2.4 mg/day, and 3 mg daily, compared to placebo (2.8 kg) and orlistat (4.1 kg). Patients taking the higher of the two doses of liraglutide (2.4 and 3 mg) lost significantly more weight than those on orlistat (6.3 kg, 7.2 kg, and 4.1 kg, respectively). However, a drawback of the drug was that at 1 year those who had reported significant nausea/vomiting episodes had the most significant weight loss at 9.2 kg while those without these side effects had a weight loss of 6.3 kg. It should be noted that the patients in this study were those without T2DM [24].

A further randomised, double-blind, controlled trial compared 3 mg of daily liraglutide to a placebo in 3731 patients without diabetes and a BMI > 30 kg/m^2 or >27 kg/m^2 if associated comorbidities. At 56 weeks, the liraglutide group had lost a mean of 8.4 ± 7.3 kg of body weight and those in the placebo group had lost a mean of 2.8 ± 6.5 kg (a difference of −5.6 kg; 95% confidence interval, −6 to −5.1, $p < 0.001$). However, a larger proportion of patients in the liraglutide group compared to the placebo group withdrew due to adverse effects (9.9% vs. 3.8%) [25]. The liraglutide group also demonstrated an improvement in cardiovascular and metabolic risk factors. Quality of life was also found to be improved in the treatment arm. A third 56-week RCT comparing weight maintenance in patients taking liraglutide compared to a placebo demonstrated maintained and further weight loss in the treatment arm [26].

Semaglutide, as stated previously, has the advantage of being a once-weekly injectable agent. The STEP 1 randomised controlled trial demonstrated a statistically significant mean weight loss compared to placebo after 68 weeks of treatment in patients without diabetes and a BMI of 30 [21]. Similar to liraglutide, the rate of discontinuation was higher in the semaglutide group (4.5% vs. 0.8%) mostly due to GI side effects. However, most patients reporting side effects in these trials had mild symptoms and resolved over time. The STEP 2 trial looked at different doses of semaglutide (1 mg and 2.4 mg once weekly) and placebo in obese patients with type 2 diabetes. The higher dose of semaglutide demonstrated the greatest reduction in weight gain [27]. Interestingly, a shorter duration of treatment as the STEP 4 trial looked at showed an increase in weight regain after switching to a placebo after 20 weeks of initial therapy [28]. Semaglutide has also been shown to reduce cardiovascular events in patients with type 2 diabetes with established cardiovascular or chronic kidney disease [29]. A recent RCT has also shown benefits of semaglutide in the reduction of cardiovascular events and deaths even in non-diabetics [30].

In both of these agents, dosing is administered in a stepwise fashion. Semaglutide dosing starts at 0.5 mg and increased at 4-week intervals until the target dose of 2.4 mg per week. Similarly, liraglutide is commenced at 1.2 mg and increased at weekly intervals to the target dose of 3 mg. The change in dose can be delayed if a patient develops side effects. The GLP1 agonists are contraindicated in pregnancy, in a patient with a history of pancreatitis, and in patients with medullary thyroid cancer of MEN 2A/2B (personal or family history). Because of the clear evidence demonstrating a weight loss benefit, concurrent diabetes treatment, and cardiometabolic benefits, the GLP-1 agonists have become first-line pharmacotherapy in obesity management. Side effects can limit use in certain patients but serious side effects are rare. Barriers to access mostly secondary to supply, cost, and reimbursement from health services have limited their access. As of January 2023, the HSE will reimburse liraglutide in 'adult patients, as an adjunct to a reduced-calorie diet and increased physical activity for weight management, with an initial body mass index of ≥35 kg/m^2 with prediabetes and high risk of cardiovascular disease', which is more stringent than the literature suggests. This leaves a gap in access to the medication for patients who may otherwise benefit. Shortages of the medication later in 2023 further complicated supply and access to the drugs.

2.3.2.2 Bupropion/Naltrexone

If the GLP-1 agonists are not tolerated, contraindicated, or cannot be accessed, then the next step of pharmacotherapy is to consider the use of bupropion–naltrexone combination. Bupropion itself acts as a noradrenaline–dopamine reuptake inhibitor and naltrexone acts as an opioid antagonist. Bupropion and naltrexone can, when used separately, be used for smoking cessation and alcohol/opiate addiction, respectively. The mechanism of action is due to the synergistic effects of the drugs acting centrally in the midbrain to decrease appetite and reduce food intake, which was discovered in animal studies [31]. A systematic review conducted in 2014 showed that in five major trials a combination of bupropion and naltrexone achieved a weight loss of at least 5%, a statistically significant difference compared to placebo, with mild side effects (mainly nausea, constipation, headache, dry mouth, vomiting, insomnia, dizziness) [32]. Nausea occurred in approximately 30% of patients vs. 5% in placebo, and constipation occurred in 14% of the treatment arm vs. 9%. A transient increase in systolic blood pressure of 1.5 mmHg and then a decrease to 1 mmHg below baseline were seen in the treatment arm [33, 34]. There was initial hesitancy to approve its use due to concern over cardiovascular effects. The full effect of the drug on the cardiovascular system has still not been fully established. This is due to a large, randomised controlled study investigating the rate of major adverse cardiovascular events (MACE) amongst overweight or obese patients using the drug being terminated early after the release of confidential interim data by the study's sponsor [35]. Interim analysis did show that the hazard ratio for MACE for the treatment arm did not exceed 2, but because of the early termination of the trial, it was not possible to fully analyse the data. Psychiatric effects of the medication should also be carefully monitored due to bupropion being theorised to cause an increase in suicidality amongst adolescents and young adults. However, a pooled analysis of five placebo-controlled trials of the combination medication in obese subjects showed no increased risk of suicidal ideation in the treatment population [36]. Contraindications of this medication include pregnancy, uncontrolled hypertension, epilepsy, eating disorders, opiate use, and severe chronic liver disease and recent mono-amine oxidase inhibitor use. The dose is gradually uptitrated over 4 weeks to 16 mg/180 mg naltrexone/bupropion twice daily, with monitoring of mood, blood pressure, and side effects being important to guide dose titration. In 2018, the NCPE recommended against reimbursement for this medication due to the uncertainty regarding cardiovascular safety and cost-effectiveness.

2.3.2.3 Phentermine–Topiramate

This combination, made up of an appetite suppressant/stimulant phentermine and an anticonvulsant topiramate, did show efficacy in achieving clinically relevant weight loss in two randomised controlled trials [37, 38]. It has been approved by the US FDA but refused by the European Medicine Agency. The FDA does not recommend the drug for patients with established cardiovascular disease or hypertension. It is also contraindicated in pregnancy due to the risk of orofacial cleft formation. Therefore, the drug is generally not prescribed in females of childbearing age, and if prescribed to this group then strict counselling, contraceptive advice, and regular pregnancy tests are essential.

Side effects in these trials included dry mouth, constipation, paraesthesia, cognitive and psychiatric side effects, as well as an increase in resting heart rate. The Committee for Medicinal Products for Human Use for the European Medicines Agency cited concerns over cardiovascular, psychiatric, cognitive, and teratogenic side effects as the main reasons for refusing its authorisation for use in the EU.

2.3.2.4 Orlistat

Another option for medical treatment are drugs that alter fat digestion, such as orlistat. This medication inhibits lipases secreted by the pancreas intra-intestinally. This leads to a decrease in fat absorption and an increase in faecal excretion. While randomised trials do indicate that orlistat is a safe and effective means of achieving weight loss, they are not as effective as other therapies (bupropion–naltrexone, semaglutide, liraglutide, phentermine–topiramate combination) [39, 40]. Studies also demonstrate benefits in blood pressure and lipid profile [41]. Unfortunately, gastrointestinal side effects such as bloating, diarrhoea, loose oily stools, and flatus occur at rates of up to 15–30% as demonstrated in a 2004 meta-analysis [42]. It can lead to a reduction in absorption of fat-soluble vitamins (A, D, E, K) and can affect warfarin metabolism [43]. A multivitamin should be co-prescribed for patients prescribed orlistat. It is also contraindicated in pregnancy or in patients suffering from malabsorption conditions, gallstones, or kidney stones.

2.3.2.5 Sympathomimetic Drugs

Finally, looking at sympathomimetic drugs such as phentermine (monotherapy), diethylpropion and benzphetamine are licensed in the United States for short-term (12 weeks) duration but are limited by side effects, including an increase in blood pressure, cardiovascular risk, insomnia, and dry mouth. Phentermine is widely prescribed in the United States due to its efficacy and low cost. New agents such as lorcaserin, a 5HT agonist acting centrally to suppress appetite, did show sustained weight loss without an increased cardiovascular risk compared to a placebo in a randomised controlled trial published in 2018 [44]. However, subsequent analyses have shown an increase in cancer risk associated with the drug, and, therefore, the FDA concluded that the risks outweigh the benefits and advised against its use [45].

2.3.3 Bariatric Surgery

Candidates for bariatric surgery include those with a BMI > 40 kg/m^2 or those 35–40 kg/m^2 with a comorbidity who have not met weight loss targets with lifestyle modification and pharmacotherapy [46]. Surgical options include a gastric band, a gastric sleeve, or gastric bypass procedures. As well as achieving a marked increase in weight loss compared to conventional therapy, bariatric surgery has also been shown to have a decrease in obesity-related morbidity and all-cause mortality at 10- to 20-year follow-ups [47]. These results have been shown to be greater still when combined with optimal lifestyle and medical therapy [48]. However, they have to be weighed against the risk of surgery itself and the side effects including mechanical and nutritional complications. Because of the extent of improvement seen with bariatric surgery, appropriate very high-risk patients should be counselled about the possibility of requiring this early on in their visits, and early surgical referral can be considered if the patient is not achieving desired outcomes on more conservative therapies.

2.4 Conclusion

To conclude, the treatment of obesity is complex. It involves a multidisciplinary approach, beginning in primary care. Prompt identification of obesity, the assessment of cardiometabolic risk factors, and other obesity-related complications are the first step of the process, with subsequent emphasis on behavioural, lifestyle, and dietary interventions. Failing this, and meeting the criteria, medical therapy could be initiated—preferably by referral to a specialised obesity clinic for a multidisciplinary assessment and initiation of more intensive lifestyle and pharmacotherapy. When a therapy is chosen, the patient's risk, comorbidities, contraindications to a specific therapy, and preferences and goals of treatment are all important to discuss at the outset of the patient's visits. Intensive lifestyle modification is the first step, but maintenance of weight loss is difficult to achieve over the long term. The preferred medical therapies are the GLP-1 agonists due to their broad range of weight and cardiometabolic benefits. Semaglutide is the desirable option due to the fact that it is injected only once weekly rather than daily. These can be limited by cost, availability, and side effects, mostly nausea/vomiting. Medications are usually discontinued if a desirable weight loss of 5% of total body weight is not achieved by 3 months. Other options include bupropion/naltrexone, phentermine/topiramate (in the United States), orlistat, or sympathomimetics; however, they do not offer as much benefit as the GLP-1 agonists and have their own side effect profiles. During medical therapy, the clinician should closely monitor heart rate, blood pressure, weight, and metabolic parameters such as lipids and blood sugars. Failure of medical therapy, in appropriate patients, should prompt surgical referral. Early surgical referral can be considered in higher risk patients deemed unlikely to benefit from more conservative approaches. At all stages, a patient-centric approach should be adopted, with aggressive co-management of cardiovascular risk factors and obesity-related complications.

References

1. World Health Organization. Obesity and overweight—WHO. https://www.Who.Int/News-Room/Fact-Sheets/Detail/Obesity-and-Overweight. 2021.
2. Sturm R, Hattori A. Morbid obesity rates continue to rise rapidly in the United States. Int J Obes. 2013;37(6):889–91.
3. Hainer V, Toplak H, Mitrakou A. Treatment modalities of obesity: what fits whom? Diabetes Care. 2008;31(Suppl 2):S269–77.
4. MacMahon S, Baigent C, Duffy S, Rodgers A, Tominaga S, Chambless L, et al. Body-mass index and cause-specific mortality in 900 000 adults: collaborative analyses of 57 prospective studies. Lancet. 2009;373(9669):1083–96.
5. Aune D, Sen A, Prasad M, Norat T, Janszky I, Tonstad S, et al. BMI and all cause mortality: systematic review and non-linear dose-response meta-analysis of 230 cohort studies with 374 million deaths among 303 million participants. BMJ (Online). 2016;353:i2156.
6. Ma C, Avenell A, Bolland M, Hudson J, Stewart F, Robertson C, et al. Effects of weight loss interventions for adults who are obese on mortality, cardiovascular disease, and cancer: systematic review and meta-analysis. BMJ. 2017;359:j4849.
7. Jensen MD, Ryan DH, Apovian CM, Ard JD, Comuzzie AG, Donato KA, et al. 2013 AHA/ACC/TOS guideline for the management of overweight and obesity in adults. Circulation. 2014;129(25 Suppl 2):S102–38.
8. Razak F, Anand SS, Shannon H, Vuksan V, Davis B, Jacobs R, et al. Defining obesity cut points in a multiethnic population. Circulation. 2007;115(16):2111–8.
9. Curry SJ, Krist AH, Owens DK, Barry MJ, Caughey AB, Davidson KW, et al. Behavioral weight loss interventions to prevent obesity-relatedmorbidity and mortality in adults US preventive services task force recommendation statement. JAMA. 2018;320(11):1163–71.
10. Bray GA, Kim KK, Wilding JPH. Obesity: a chronic relapsing progressive disease process. A position statement of the World Obesity Federation. Obes Rev. 2017;18(7):715–23.
11. Garvey WT, Mechanick JI, Brett EM, Garber AJ, Hurley DL, Jastreboff AM, et al. American association of clinical endocrinologists and American college of endocrinology comprehensive clinical practice guidelines for medical care of patients with obesity. Endocr Pract. 2016;22(Suppl 3):1–203.
12. Tsai AG, Wadden TA. The evolution of very-low-calorie diets: an update and meta-analysis. Obesity. 2006;14(8):1283–93.

13. Piercy KL, Troiano RP, Ballard RM, Carlson SA, Fulton JE, Galuska DA, et al. The physical activity guidelines for Americans. JAMA. 2018;320(19):2020–8.
14. Blüher M. Obesity: global epidemiology and pathogenesis. Nat Rev Endocrinol. 2019;15(5):288–98.
15. Leslie WS, Hankey CR, Lean MEJ. Weight gain as an adverse effect of some commonly prescribed drugs: a systematic review. QJM. 2007;100(7):395–404.
16. Apovian CM, Aronne LJ, Bessesen DH, McDonnell ME, Murad MH, Pagotto U, et al. Pharmacological management of obesity: an endocrine society clinical practice guideline. J Clin Endocrinol Metab. 2015;100(2):342–62.
17. Khera R, Murad MH, Chandar AK, Dulai PS, Wang Z, Prokop LJ, et al. Association of pharmacological treatments for obesity with weight loss and adverse events a systematic review and meta-analysis. JAMA. 2016;315(22):2424–34.
18. Bray GA, Frühbeck G, Ryan DH, Wilding JPH. Management of obesity. Lancet. 2016;387(10031):1947–56.
19. Ara R, Blake L, Gray L, Hernández M, Crowther M, Dunkley A, et al. What is the clinical effectiveness and cost-effectiveness of using drugs in treating obese patients in primary care? A systematic review. Health Technol Assess (Rockv). 2012;16(5):iii–xiv.
20. Nuffer WA, Trujillo JM. Liraglutide: a new option for the treatment of obesity. Pharmacother apy. 2015;35(10):926–34.
21. Wilding JPH, Batterham RL, Calanna S, Davies M, Van Gaal LF, Lingvay I, et al. Once-weekly semaglutide in adults with overweight or obesity. N Engl J Med. 2021;384(11):989–1002.
22. Wadden TA, Hollander P, Klein S, Niswender K, Woo V, Hale PM, et al. Weight maintenance and additional weight loss with liraglutide after low-calorie-diet-induced weight loss: the SCALE maintenance randomized study. Int J Obes. 2013;37(11):1443–51.
23. Overgaard RV, Petri KC, Jacobsen LV, Jensen CB. Liraglutide 3.0 mg for weight management: a population pharmacokinetic analysis. Clin Pharmacokinet. 2016;55(11):1413–22.
24. Astrup A, Rössner S, Van Gaal L, Rissanen A, Niskanen L, Al Hakim M, et al. Effects of liraglutide in the treatment of obesity: a randomised, double-blind, placebo-controlled study. Lancet. 2009;374(9701):1606–16.
25. Pi-Sunyer X, Astrup A, Fujioka K, Greenway F, Halpern A, Krempf M, et al. A randomized, controlled trial of 3.0 mg of liraglutide in weight management. N Engl J Med. 2015;373(1):11–22.
26. Wadden TA, Hollander P, Klein S, Niswender K, Woo V, Hale PM, et al. Weight maintenance and additional weight loss with liraglutide after low-calorie-diet-induced weight loss: the SCALE maintenance randomized study. Int J Obes. 2015;39:187. Erratum
27. Davies M, Færch L, Jeppesen OK, Pakseresht A, Pedersen SD, Perreault L, et al. Semaglutide 2·4 mg once a week in adults with overweight or obesity, and type 2 diabetes (STEP 2): a randomised, double-blind, double-dummy, placebo-controlled, phase 3 trial. Lancet. 2021;397(10278):971–84.
28. Rubino D, Abrahamsson N, Davies M, Hesse D, Greenway FL, Jensen C, et al. Effect of continued weekly subcutaneous Semaglutide vs placebo on weight loss maintenance in adults with overweight or obesity: the STEP 4 randomized clinical trial. JAMA. 2021;325(14):1414–25.
29. Marso SP, Eliaschewitz FG, Jódar E, Leiter LA, Hansen O, Holst AG, for the SUSTAIN-6 Investigators, et al. Semaglutide and cardiovascular outcomes in patients with type 2 diabetes. N Engl J Med. 2016;375:1834–44.
30. Lincoff AM, Brown-Frandsen K, Colhoun HM, Deanfield J, Emerson SS, Esbjerg S, et al. Semaglutide and cardiovascular outcomes in obesity without diabetes. N Engl J Med. 2023;389(24):2221–32.
31. Greenway FL, Whitehouse MJ, Guttadauria M, Anderson JW, Atkinson RL, Fujioka K, et al. Rational design of a combination medication for the treatment of obesity. Obesity. 2009;17(1):30–9.
32. Caixàs A, Albert L, Capel I, Rigla M. Naltrexone sustained-release/bupropion sustained-release for the management of obesity: review of the data to date. Drug Des Devel Ther. 2014;8:1419–27.

33. Greenway FL, Fujioka K, Plodkowski RA, Mudaliar S, Guttadauria M, Erickson J, et al. Effect of naltrexone plus bupropion on weight loss in overweight and obese adults (COR-I): a multicentre, randomised, double-blind, placebo-controlled, phase 3 trial. Lancet. 2010;376(9741):595–605.
34. Apovian CM, Aronne L, Rubino D, Still C, Wyatt H, Burns C, et al. A randomized, phase 3 trial of naltrexone SR/bupropion SR on weight and obesity-related risk factors (COR-II). Obesity. 2013;21(5):935–43.
35. Nissen SE, Wolski KE, Prcela L, Wadden T, Buse JB, Bakris G, et al. Effect of naltrexone-bupropion on major adverse cardiovascular events in overweight and obese patients with cardiovascular risk factors: a randomized clinical trial. JAMA. 2016;315(10):990–1004.
36. Pi-Sunyer X, Apovian CM, McElroy SL, Dunayevich E, Acevedo LM, Greenway FL. Psychiatric adverse events and effects on mood with prolonged-release naltrexone/bupropion combination therapy: a pooled analysis. Int J Obes. 2019;43(10):2085–94.
37. Gadde KM, Allison DB, Ryan DH, Peterson CA, Troupin B, Schwiers ML, et al. Effects of low-dose, controlled-release, phentermine plus topiramate combination on weight and associated comorbidities in overweight and obese adults (CONQUER): a randomised, placebo-controlled, phase 3 trial. Lancet. 2011;377(9774):1341–52.
38. Allison DB, Gadde KM, Garvey WT, Peterson CA, Schwiers ML, Najarian T, et al. Controlled-release phentermine/topiramate in severely obese adults: a randomized controlled trial (EQUIP). Obesity. 2012;20(2):330–42.
39. Sjöström L, Rissanen A, Andersen T, Boldrin M, Golay A, Koppeschaar HPF, et al. Randomised placebo-controlled trial of orlistat for weight loss and prevention of weight regain in obese patients. Lancet. 1998;352(9123):167–72.
40. Davidson MH, Hauptman J, DiGirolamo M, Foreyt JP, Halsted CH, Heber D, et al. Weight control and risk factor reduction in obese subjects treated for 2 years with orlistat: a randomized controlled trial. JAMA. 1999;281(3):235–42.
41. Siebenhofer A, Winterholer S, Jeitler K, Horvath K, Berghold A, Krenn C, et al. Long-term effects of weight-reducing drugs in people with hypertension. Cochrane Database Syst Rev. 2021;1(1):CD007654.
42. Padwal RS, Rucker D, Li SK, Curioni C, Lau DCW. Long-term pharmacotherapy for obesity and overweight. Cochrane Database Syst Rev. 2003;335(7631):1194–9.
43. MacWalter RS, Fraser HW, Armstrong KM, Rivera-Miranda G, Dion P. Orlistat enhances warfarin effect. Ann Pharmacother. 2003;37(4):510–2.
44. Bohula EA, Wiviott SD, McGuire DK, Inzucchi SE, Kuder J, Im K, et al. Cardiovascular safety of lorcaserin in overweight or obese patients. N Engl J Med. 2018;379(12):1107–17.
45. Sharretts J, Galescu O, Gomatam S, Andraca-Carrera E, Hampp C, Yanoff L. Cancer risk associated with lorcaserin—the FDA's review of the CAMELLIA-TIMI 61 trial. N Engl J Med. 2020;383(11):1000–2.
46. Rubino F, Nathan DM, Eckel RH, Schauer PR, Alberti KGMM, Zimmet PZ, et al. Metabolic surgery in the treatment algorithm for type 2 diabetes: a joint statement by international diabetes organizations. Diabetes Care. 2016;39(6):861–77.
47. Sjöström L. Review of the key results from the Swedish Obese Subjects (SOS) trial—a prospective controlled intervention study of bariatric surgery. J Intern Med. 2013;273(3):219–34.
48. Schauer PR, Bhatt DL, Kirwan JP, Wolski K, Aminian A, Brethauer SA, et al. Bariatric surgery versus intensive medical therapy for diabetes—5-year outcomes. N Engl J Med. 2017;376(7):641–51.

Surgical Treatment of Obesity

3

Orlaith Kelly, Bisola Salaja, Aisling O'Byrne,
and Helen Heneghan

3.1 Introduction

The rising prevalence of obesity and high numbers of non-responders to non-surgical weight management programmes have led to the evolution of surgical treatments for obesity [1–3]. The surgical management of obesity can be referred to as obesity, bariatric, or metabolic surgery. Whilst these treatments were initially conceived purely for weight loss, bariatric surgery has since evolved into a treatment for health gain. An abundance of evidence now demonstrates that bariatric surgery is not only superior to usual medical care for weight loss, but more importantly translates into several health benefits including improved glycaemic control and reductions in morbidity and mortality from cardiovascular disease and cancer [4–9].

Obesity is associated with several complications including heart disease, stroke, type 2 diabetes mellitus, osteoarthritis, many cancers, depression, liver disease, and obstructive sleep apnoea [1]. Bariatric surgery can cause significant improvements in most, if not all, of these conditions and can even put many into remission. In addition to weight loss and improvement in medical comorbidities, patient-reported

O. Kelly (✉)
Royal College of Surgeons Ireland, RCSI, Dublin, Ireland
e-mail: kellyo6@tcd.ie

B. Salaja
University College Hospital/Merlin Park Regional Hospital, Galway, Ireland

A. O'Byrne
Trinity College Dublin, TCD, Dublin, Ireland
e-mail: obyrnea@tcd.ie

H. Heneghan
St. Vincent's University Hospital, Dublin, Ireland
e-mail: Helen.heneghan@ucd.ie

J. M. O´Byrne et al. (eds.), *Musculoskeletal Disease and Obesity*,
https://doi.org/10.1007/978-3-031-63310-2_3

outcome measures such as quality-of-life improvements are significant. Also, 95% of patients who undergo bariatric surgery will report an improvement in their quality of life within 6 months of the procedure [2]. Obesity is known to reduce average life expectancy by approximately 5–10 years. Data from the Swedish Obese Subjects (SOS) study shows that bariatric surgery can prolong life by at least 3 years compared to those treated with non-surgical care [3].

3.2 Eligibility for Bariatric Surgery

The eligibility criteria for bariatric surgery that are still widely used today were established in 1991 by the National Institute of Health (NIH) [4]. As per these criteria, patients are considered eligible for bariatric surgery if they have a body mass index (BMI) of over 35 kg/m^2 in the presence of an obesity-related comorbidity such as diabetes mellitus, hypertension, hypercholesterolaemia, or obstructive sleep apnoea. Patients with a BMI of 40 kg/m^2 or more are also considered eligible, regardless of comorbidities.

The understanding of the disease of obesity and benefits of bariatric surgery has grown significantly since the NIH guidelines were published 30 years ago. The American Society for Metabolic and Bariatric Surgery (ASMBS) and the International Federation for the Surgery of Obesity and Metabolic Disorders (IFSO) have recently published new recommendations for eligibility criteria for bariatric surgery [5]. They recommend bariatric surgery for individuals with BMI ≥35 kg/m^2, regardless of comorbidities as well as in patients with type 2 diabetes mellitus and BMI ≥30 kg/m^2. According to ASMBS and IFSO, bariatric surgery should also be considered in patients with a BMI of 30–34.9 kg/m^2 who cannot achieve a desirable or sustained weight loss, or improvement in medical comorbidities, using non-surgical options. They suggest that there is no upper age limit for bariatric surgery and that consideration for bariatric surgery in older patients should involve careful assessment of comorbidities and frailty.

It is important that patients have made previous attempts at weight loss for a minimum time period of 6 months. It is also considered essential that patients accept the risks associated with these surgical procedures and agree to comply with lifelong lifestyle changes as well as with regular postoperative follow-up as per international guidelines [5]. There are a number of contraindications to bariatric surgery. These include a person's inability to comply with nutritional requirements postoperatively, patients with active/untreated eating disorders, severe coagulopathy, major depression or psychosis, current drug or alcohol dependence or misuse, and severe cardiac disease with prohibitive anaesthetic risks.

Input from a multidisciplinary team, including both a registered dietician and mental health provider, is essential prior to undergoing bariatric surgery. A nutritional assessment is important in ensuring that any maladaptive eating behaviours are identified and addressed. Identifying and correcting micronutrient deficiencies preoperatively, as well as preparing the patient for expected dietary changes following bariatric surgery, are part of the essential role of the dietician in the multidisciplinary team assessment. Psychological evaluation preoperatively is imperative to optimise surgical outcomes and ensure that patients have the ability to cope with the challenges of undergoing surgery, changes in body image and lifestyle that are required following bariatric surgery [5].

Bariatric surgery procedures aim to induce weight loss and metabolic health gain. This was thought to be achieved via two mechanisms: malabsorption, restriction, or a combination of both:

- Malabsorption
  - Decreases absorption of nutrients by shortening the absorptive length of the small intestine, either by bypassing the small bowel absorptive surface area or diverting biliopancreatic secretions that facilitate absorption.
    For example, jejunoileal bypass; biliopancreatic diversion.
- Restriction
  - Limits caloric intake by reducing the capacity of the stomach via resection, creation of a proximal gastric outlet or bypass.
    For example, laparoscopic-adjustable gastric banding, sleeve gastrectomy.
- Combination of restriction and malabsorption
  - Roux-en-Y gastric bypass: a small gastric pouch limits oral intake while reconfiguration of the small bowel results in mild malabsorption, beneficial gut hormonal change, and dumping physiology.

3.3 Bariatric Surgery Procedures

Sleeve gastrectomy, Roux-en-Y gastric bypass (RYGB), biliopancreatic diversion (BPD) with or without duodenal switch (DS), and gastric banding (GB) are the most commonly performed bariatric procedures worldwide at present. These operations have traditionally been categorised as restrictive (gastric band and sleeve), malabsorptive (BPD, DS), or combined restrictive and malabsorptive (RYGB) procedures. However, this classification is unscientific and an increasing body of literature demonstrates that mechanisms other than restriction and malabsorption are at play. It has emerged that procedure effects are largely determined by visceral signals which occur as a result of anatomic alterations to the gut [10, 11]. It is these visceral signals and other endocrine changes (the so-called weight-independent mechanisms) which are largely responsible for the effects of bariatric surgery. Gastric banding and sleeve gastrectomy only alter stomach anatomy, whereas RYGB and BPD involve anatomical alterations of both the stomach and the small bowel. The mechanism of action of each procedure results in unique outcomes and can give rise to a constellation of procedure-specific risks, benefits, and limitations, as outlined below.

All of these procedures are performed laparoscopically, with rates of conversion to open surgery now less than 1%. Enhanced recovery after surgery (ERAS) protocols are widely used by bariatric surgery providers to improve surgical outcomes. These protocols include a bundle of measures preoperatively, intraoperatively, and postoperatively that have been shown to decrease complications, operative time, and length of hospital stay [12].

3.4 Roux-en-Y Gastric Bypass

Often considered to be the gold-standard bariatric procedure, the RYGB involves creating a small proximal gastric pouch (30–50 ml in volume), following which the small intestine is divided 50–100 cm distal to the ligament of Treitz in order to create the biliopancreatic limb and the Roux limb. The Roux limb is connected to the proximal gastric pouch, and the biliopancreatic limb is connected to the Roux limb approximately 100–150 cm distal to the gastrojejunal anastomosis.

This anatomical rearrangement has a number of effects:

- The new gastric pouch is only able to hold a small amount of food, resulting in feeling full after consuming only a very small amount (early satiety).
- Ghrelin is a peptide hormone secreted in the foregut (stomach and duodenum) that stimulates appetite. After gastric bypass, the secretion of Ghrelin is inhibited due to the foregut bypass.
- Leptin, glucagon-like peptide-1 (GLP-1), and cholecystokinin (CCK) levels are increased following RYGB, promoting an anorectic state.
- Changes in intestinal nutrient-sensing mechanisms improve insulin sensitivity.
- Bile acid absorption and the gut microbiome are altered.
- The anatomy of the gastrojejunostomy (connection between stomach and jejunum) and intestinal bypass is associated with dumping physiology, leading to nausea, diaphoresis, light-headedness, abdominal pain, and diarrhoea when a high-sugar and/or high-fat meal is ingested. This may result in negative conditioning against consumption of a high-sugar and high-fat diet postoperatively.

It is expected that patients will lose approximately 25–30% of their preop total body weight in the first 2 years after RYGB, and long-term total body weight loss is approximately 25%. In terms of comorbidities, RYGB has been shown to induce remission of type 2 diabetes mellitus in up to 80% of patients at 2 years postoperatively and up to 50% at 12 years postoperatively [13–15] An improvement in reflux symptoms in up to 56% of patients that have undergone RYGB has been demonstrated, and so this procedure is considered a better procedure for patients with pre-existing gastro-oesophageal reflux compared to sleeve gastrectomy [16].

Laparoscopic RYGB is associated with a 30-day mortality of 1 in 1000, which is similar to the mortality rates of some of the most commonly performed surgical procedures such as laparoscopic cholecystectomy [17]. The leading cause of death in the 90 days after bariatric surgery is thromboembolic disease. Complication rates vary from 1 to 20% in the literature [18]. Specific concerns after RYGB include postoperative bleeding, staple line or anastomotic leak, anastomotic ulcer and/or stricture, and internal hernia. The leak rate is approximately 1% in high-volume bariatric centres [19]. The most common complication after RYGB is iron deficiency anaemia, which is usually minor and treated with additional iron supplementation.

As with all bariatric procedures, patients require regular lifelong monitoring of vitamins and minerals and routine supplementation of the same postoperatively.

3.5 Sleeve Gastrectomy

Sleeve gastrectomy is the most commonly performed bariatric procedure worldwide at present [7]. Similar to gastric bypass, it is effective for both weight loss and health gain. Weight loss is achieved through both mechanical (restrictive) and endocrine mechanisms. The sleeve gastrectomy is also performed laparoscopically and involves resecting the greater curvature of the stomach, leaving behind a tubular stomach. Removal of the gastric fundus is largely responsible for the major endocrine changes observed after sleeve gastrectomy including postprandial increases in intestinal hormones such as glucagon-like peptide (GLP)-1 and peptide YY (PYY), as well as decreases in fasting ghrelin levels, resulting in patients feeling less hungry and more full [8, 9].

The laparoscopic sleeve gastrectomy is considered slightly less effective but also less morbid than RYBG. Short- to medium-term outcomes show total weight loss of approximately 20–25% of preoperative weight and long-term total body weight loss of approximately 20% [20]. There is a higher risk of weight regain after sleeve gastrectomy compared to RYGB. The rates of weight regain vary widely in the literature, from 14% to 37% at 7 years postoperatively [10].

The risk of 30-day mortality after sleeve gastrectomy is approximately 1 in 1000, comparable to that after RYGB [11]. Morbidity rates are low and vary from 0% to 17.5% in the literature [18]. Specific concerns after sleeve gastrectomy include staple line bleeding, staple line leak and gastro-oesophageal reflux disease. The leak rate is approximately 1–2% [21]. A meta-analysis of 46 studies found that 19% of patients had worsening reflux and 23% developed de novo reflux after sleeve gastrectomy. The long-term prevalence of oesophagitis and Barrett's oesophagus after sleeve gastrectomy was 28% and 8%, respectively. Also, 4% of patients required conversion to RYGB due to severe reflux [22].

3.6 Gastric Banding

Gastric banding involves placement of an adjustable soft silicone band around the proximal stomach, just 2 cm below the oesophagogastric junction. The gastric band is a soft silicone ring which is connected by tubing to an infusion port which is placed in subcutaneous tissue. Saline can be injected into the port, resulting in a reduction in the diameter of the band and increased restriction. The goal of adjusting the band is to restrict the patient's food intake to approximately one cup of solid food per meal and result in satiety for at least 2 h following a meal. Historically, it was the most popular surgical procedure for weight loss but is now performed much less frequently (approximately 6% of all procedures). Its decline is largely due to its poor long-term efficacy in terms of weight loss and health gain. Failure rates of gastric banding approach 40% at 7 years postoperatively. A procedure is considered to have failed if there has been insufficient weight loss or a major complication necessitating band removal, with or without conversion to another bariatric procedure [6]. It is also important to note that gastric banding has little effect on gut hormone secretion and visceral signalling, unlike other bariatric procedures. Procedure-specific complications include slippage of the band, band erosion into the stomach, gastroesophageal reflux, and oesophageal dysmotility.

3.7 Biliopancreatic Diversion with Duodenal Switch (BPD/DS)

BPD-DS involves, firstly, creating a sleeve gastrectomy, then creating an intestinal bypass involving a long Roux limb and short common channel (100–150 cm). It is a malabsorptive procedure that leads to significant weight loss. The expected total body weight loss 2 years postop is approximately 35–40%. The mechanisms of action of a BPD-DS mirror those of RYGB, but are more exaggerated. Whilst it is a very effective procedure for weight loss and metabolic health improvements, it can lead to malnutrition due to malabsorption, particularly of fat-soluble vitamins (vitamins A, D, E, K).

3.8 Late Complications of Bariatric Surgery

Long-term complications of bariatric surgery are often unique to the specific procedure, but there are a number of general issues relevant to all bariatric procedures. Special attention must always be given to the nutritional status of patients following bariatric procedures, particularly after malabsorptive operations. Deficiency of essential vitamins and minerals is more common following RYGB and BPD-DS, and on very rare occasions may be life threatening, as with thiamine deficiency-related encephalopathy. It is essential that the multidisciplinary team managing bariatric patients be mindful of the micronutrient deficiencies and dietary supplementation following these procedures.

Lifelong supplementation of vitamins D and B12, folic acid, iron, and calcium, among others, is recommended [23]. Scheduled surveillance of these nutritional parameters by blood tests is recommended on a regular basis, at 3-month intervals for the first postoperative year, 6-monthly for the second postoperative year, and annually thereafter [23].

Another diet-related problem after bariatric surgery, specifically after gastric bypass and BPD-DS, is dumping syndrome which occurs shortly after eating in approximately 50% of patients after RYGB at some stage postoperatively [19]. It is characterised by symptoms such as nausea, tremors, sweating, diarrhoea, dizziness, flushing, tachycardia, and occasionally syncope, resulting from the ingestion of food containing large quantities of refined sugars (high glycaemic index foods) and from food eaten too quickly. Whilst this was initially considered a desirable deterrent from such behaviours, particularly in patients who are partial to sweet foods, no association between symptoms and weight loss has ever been shown. Moreover, dumping syndrome can be very problematic in approximately 1% of patients [19]. Another group of patients suffer from postprandial hyperinsulinemic hypoglycaemia (PPH) with neuroglycopenia, often called 'late dumping', potentially due to changes in the gut hormonal milieu [19]. Strict dietary alteration is required to manage this, with patients advised to eat more low glycaemic index carbohydrates and protein, and to avoid any medium or high glycaemic index carbohydrates. Patients whose symptoms do not respond to dietary interventions may require a trial of diazoxide, octreotide, or calcium-channel antagonists to ameliorate the debilitating symptoms of PPH [19], while GLP-1 analogues have also recently been shown to have benefits.Other late complications of bariatric surgery relate to the significant weight loss it induces. These include gallstone formation, hair thinning, and excess skin [24, 25]. The latter can significantly affect body image and satisfaction with the surgical outcome. In addition to the aesthetic problem, it can lead to functional problems, dermatoses, and difficulties in maintaining satisfactory personal hygiene. Treatment of loose/excess skin is mainly with body contouring surgery, for which there are guidelines from the international Plastic and Reconstructive Surgery associations [26, 27]. Another troublesome complication after bariatric surgery is nonspecific abdominal pain which can occur in 5–10% of patients. The diagnosis and treatment of this nonspecific pain can be very challenging as it is important to try to avoid opiate use.

3.9 Adverse Effects of Bariatric Surgery on Bone Health

Bariatric surgery-induced bone loss has gained much attention in recent years. Bone mineral density has been shown to reduce following bariatric surgery by approximately 5–14% from baseline [28, 29]. Bone loss in this setting appears multifactorial and causes include nutrient deficiencies, changes in both gut and gonadal hormones, mechanical unloading, loss of lean mass, and increased bone marrow fat. Deficiencies in calcium and vitamin D can lead to secondary hyperparathyroidism and excessive bone resorption. Mechanical unloading contributes to bone loss through the inhibition of bone formation and stimulation of bone resorption [28].

It is important that bone health is prioritised following bariatric surgery. This requires a multidisciplinary approach, including the medical team, dietician, and physiotherapist. It is important that patients are screened preoperatively for deficiencies in bone health, and, as previously described, patients are discharged home following their surgery with appropriate nutritional supplements. The British

Obesity and Metabolic Surgery Society (BOMSS) provides recommendations for the monitoring and supplementation of minerals and vitamins. Vitamin D3 supplementation should aim to achieve a serum 25-hydroxyvitamin D level of 75 mmol/L or higher. This may require 2000–4000 IU of oral vitamin D3 per day following malabsorptive bariatric procedures and 1200–1500 mg calcium per day is recommended between dietary calcium and supplementation [30]. It is recommended that patients undergo a preoperative dual-energy X-ray absorptiometry (DEXA) scan, and that this is repeated every 2 years following malabsorptive procedures [31]. The physiotherapist plays an essential role in ensuring that patients partake in weight-bearing exercise postoperatively in an effort to minimise reductions in bone mineral density.

3.10 Summary

In addition to achieving substantial and durable weight loss, bariatric surgery is associated with favourable metabolic effects far beyond those achieved by lifestyle modifications and pharmacological treatments. Perioperative morbidity and mortality have decreased significantly over the last two decades such that the safety profile of bariatric surgery is now as favourable as commonly performed general surgery procedures, such as cholecystectomy. Bariatric surgery is also associated with significant improvements in long-term mortality and longevity. Much of the improvement in perioperative morbidity and mortality can be attributed to advances in laparoscopic surgery, ERAS protocols, as well as the establishment of high-volume centres of excellence and required outcome reporting. The current extensive evidence demonstrating the safety and efficacy of bariatric surgery supports it as the current standard of care for the treatment of severe obesity and its related complications.

References

1. Malnick SD, Knobler H. The medical complications of obesity. QJM. 2006;99(9):565–79.
2. Castanha CR, Tcbc-Pe ÁABF, Castanha AR, Belo G, Lacerda RMR, Vilar L. Evaluation of quality of life, weight loss and comorbidities of patients undergoing bariatric surgery. Rev Col Bras Cir. 2018;45(3):e1864.
3. Carlsson LMS, Sjöholm K, Jacobson P, Andersson-Assarsson JC, Svensson P-A, Taube M, et al. Life expectancy after bariatric surgery in the Swedish obese subjects study. N Engl J Med. 2020;383(16):1535–43.
4. Gastrointestinal surgery for severe obesity. National Institutes of Health consensus development conference statement. Am J Clin Nutr. 1992;55(2):615S–9S.
5. Eisenberg D, Shikora SA, Aarts E, Aminian A, Angrisani L, Cohen RV, et al. 2022 American Society for Metabolic and Bariatric Surgery (ASMBS) and International Federation for the Surgery of Obesity and Metabolic Disorders (IFSO): indications for metabolic and bariatric surgery. Surg Obes Relat Dis. 2022;18(12):1345–56.
6. Suter M, Calmes JM, Paroz A, Giusti V. A 10-year experience with laparoscopic gastric banding for morbid obesity: high long-term complication and failure rates. Obes Surg. 2006;16(7):829–35.

7. Ponce J, DeMaria EJ, Nguyen NT, Hutter M, Sudan R, Morton JM. American Society for Metabolic and Bariatric Surgery estimation of bariatric surgery procedures in 2015 and surgeon workforce in the United States. Surg Obes Relat Dis. 2016;12(9):1637–9.
8. McCarty TR, Jirapinyo P, Thompson CC. Effect of sleeve gastrectomy on ghrelin, GLP-1, PYY, and GIP gut hormones: a systematic review and meta-analysis. Ann Surg. 2020;272(1):72–80.
9. Ionut V, Bergman RN. Mechanisms responsible for excess weight loss after bariatric surgery. J Diabetes Sci Technol. 2011;5(5):1263–82.
10. Clapp B, Wynn M, Martyn C, Foster C, O'Dell M, Tyroch A. Long term (7 or more years) outcomes of the sleeve gastrectomy: a meta-analysis. Surg Obes Relat Dis. 2018;14(6):741–7.
11. Young MT, Gebhart A, Phelan MJ, Nguyen NT. Use and outcomes of laparoscopic sleeve gastrectomy vs laparoscopic gastric bypass: analysis of the American College of Surgeons NSQIP. J Am Coll Surg. 2015;220(5):880–5.
12. Kearns E, O'Reilly P, Lawton C, McMackin T, Heneghan H, Fearon N. Enhanced recovery after bariatric surgery: clinical outcomes in a tertiary referral bariatric centre. Mesentery Peritoneum. 2020;4:AB058.
13. Buchwald H, Estok R, Fahrbach K, Banel D, Jensen MD, Pories WJ, et al. Weight and type 2 diabetes after bariatric surgery: systematic review and meta-analysis. Am J Med. 2009;122(3):248–56.e5.
14. Adams TD, Davidson LE, Litwin SE, Kim J, Kolotkin RL, Nanjee MN, et al. Weight and metabolic outcomes 12 years after gastric bypass. N Engl J Med. 2017;377(12):1143–55.
15. Al SJ. STAMPEDE: bariatric surgery gains more evidence based support. Glob Cardiol Sci Pract. 2014;2014(1):45–8. https://doi.org/10.5339/gcsp.2014.8.
16. Pallati PK, Shaligram A, Shostrom VK, Oleynikov D, McBride CL, Goede MR. Improvement in gastroesophageal reflux disease symptoms after various bariatric procedures: review of the Bariatric Outcomes Longitudinal Database. Surg Obes Relat Dis. 2014;10(3):502–7.
17. DeMaria EJ, Pate V, Warthen M, Winegar DA. Baseline data from American Society for Metabolic and Bariatric Surgery-designated Bariatric Surgery Centers of Excellence using the Bariatric Outcomes Longitudinal Database. Surg Obes Relat Dis. 2010;6(4):347–55.
18. Fischer L, Hildebrandt C, Bruckner T, Kenngott H, Linke GR, Gehrig T, et al. Excessive weight loss after sleeve gastrectomy: a systematic review. Obes Surg. 2012;22(5):721–31.
19. Jacobsen HJ, Nergard BJ, Leifsson BG, Frederiksen SG, Agajahni E, Ekelund M, et al. Management of suspected anastomotic leak after bariatric laparoscopic Roux-en-y gastric bypass. Br J Surg. 2014;101(4):417–23.
20. Himpens J, Dobbeleir J, Peeters G. Long-term results of laparoscopic sleeve gastrectomy for obesity. Ann Surg. 2010;252(2)
21. Aurora AR, Khaitan L, Saber AA. Sleeve gastrectomy and the risk of leak: a systematic analysis of 4,888 patients. Surg Endosc. 2012;26(6):1509–15.
22. Yeung KTD, Penney N, Ashrafian L, Darzi A, Ashrafian H. Does sleeve gastrectomy expose the distal esophagus to severe reflux?: a systematic review and meta-analysis. Ann Surg. 2020;271(2):257–65.
23. Zhang W, Fan M, Wang C, Mahawar K, Parmar C, Chen W, et al. Hair loss after metabolic and bariatric surgery: a systematic review and meta-analysis. Obes Surg. 2021;31(6):2649–59.
24. Robert M, Espalieu P, Pelascini E, Caiazzo R, Sterkers A, Khamphommala L, et al. Efficacy and safety of one anastomosis gastric bypass versus Roux-en-Y gastric bypass for obesity (YOMEGA): a multicentre, randomised, open-label, non-inferiority trial. Lancet (British edition). 2019;393(10178):1299–309.
25. Poljo A, Pentsch A, Raab S, Klugsberger B, Shamiyeh A. Incidence of dumping syndrome after sleeve gastrectomy, Roux-en-Y gastric bypass and one-anastomosis gastric bypass. J Metab Bariatr Surg. 2021;10(1):23–31.
26. Talha A, Abdelbaki T, Farouk A, Hasouna E, Azzam E, Shehata G. Cholelithiasis after bariatric surgery, incidence, and prophylaxis: randomized controlled trial. Surg Endosc. 2020;34(12):5331–7.

27. Soldin M, Mughal M, Al-Hadithy N. National commissioning guidelines: body contouring surgery after massive weight loss. J Plast Reconstr Aesthet Surg. 2014;67(8):1076–81.
28. Saad R, Habli D, El Sabbagh R, Chakhtoura M. Bone health following bariatric surgery: an update. J Clin Densitom. 2020;23(2):165–81.
29. Liu C, Wu D, Zhang JF, Xu D, Xu WF, Chen Y, et al. Changes in bone metabolism in morbidly obese patients after bariatric surgery: a meta-analysis. Obes Surg. 2016;26(1):91–7.
30. O'Kane M, Parretti HM, Pinkney J, Welbourn R, Hughes CA, Mok J, et al. British Obesity and Metabolic Surgery Society Guidelines on perioperative and postoperative biochemical monitoring and micronutrient replacement for patients undergoing bariatric surgery—2020 update. Obes Rev. 2020;21(11):e13087.
31. Mechanick JI, Apovian C, Brethauer S, Timothy Garvey W, Joffe AM, Kim J, et al. Clinical practice guidelines for the perioperative nutrition, metabolic, and nonsurgical support of patients undergoing bariatric procedures—2019 update: cosponsored by American Association of Clinical Endocrinologists/American College of Endocrinology, The Obesity Society, American Society for Metabolic and Bariatric Surgery, Obesity Medicine Association, and American Society of Anesthesiologists. Obesity. 2020;28(4):O1–O58.
32. le Roux CW, Heneghan HM. Bariatric surgery for obesity. Med Clin North Am. 2018;102(1):165–82.

Obesity and Trauma

4

Michael Hanlon, Olivia Horner, Fred Kenny, and Barry O'Neill

4.1 Introduction

When we hear the word 'malnutrition', we often think of individuals who are undernourished and thin. However, the American Society for Parenteral and Enteral Nutrition (ASPEN) defines malnutrition as a state of nutrition in which a combination of varying degrees of overnutrition or undernutrition has led to changes in body composition and diminished function [1]. Obese individuals are, therefore, by definition, malnourished. Obesity is defined by the World Health Organization (WHO) as an abnormal or excessive fat accumulation that may impair health. More specifically, obesity is defined as a body mass index (BMI) of greater than 30. BMI is calculated by dividing a person's weight (in kilograms) by the square of their height (in metres). The accepted clinical interpretations of the calculated BMI are shown in Table 4.1.

Table 4.1 Clinical interpretations of BMI

BMI (kg/m^2)	Interpretation
18.5–24.9	Normal weight
25–29.9	Overweight
30–34.9	Obese
35.0–39.9	Extremely obese
>40	Morbidly obese

M. Hanlon · F. Kenny (✉)
National Orthopaedic Hospital Cappagh, Dublin, Ireland

O. Horner
Tallaght University Hospital, Dublin, Ireland
e-mail: hornero@tcd.ie

B. O'Neill
Sligo Regional University Hospital, Sligo, Ireland

J. M. O´Byrne et al. (eds.), *Musculoskeletal Disease and Obesity*,
https://doi.org/10.1007/978-3-031-63310-2_4

Since 1975, obesity has almost tripled within the worldwide population [2]. It is estimated that there are 650 million obese adults worldwide, and by 2025 this figure is expected to have surpassed 1 billion people [2]. This growing social problem, and its adverse effects on health, has led to significant efforts by healthcare systems all over the world to educate individuals and reduce the burden of obesity on healthcare provision. It is known that obesity can have a significant adverse effect on various organs and systems within the body [3]. It is known to be associated with reduced life expectancy, cardiac disease, diabetes mellitus, and psychological dysfunction. It is for this reason that many surgeons now insist upon obese patients losing weight prior to elective procedures in order to reduce the potential for intraoperative and postoperative complications associated with obesity.

Trauma surgeons do not have this opportunity to address obesity preoperatively. Individual trauma results from an event, series of events, or set of circumstances that are experienced by an individual as physically or emotionally harmful or threatening and that can have lasting adverse effects on the individual's functioning and physical, social, and emotional well-being. For the remainder of this discussion, we are going to assume that the word 'trauma' refers to a single incident that causes immediate physical harm to the individual involved, often including a fracture (a fracture is defined as a soft-tissue injury complicated by the presence of a broken bone). We will assume that the physical harm (injury) requires immediate attention and there is no opportunity to address the individual's obesity prior to commencing treatment of the injury. We therefore have to look at obesity in trauma from a slightly different perspective than obesity in elective orthopaedic surgery. We need to know which complications are more likely to occur in obese patients who have sustained a traumatic injury in order to anticipate these complications and address them prospectively where possible.

The BMI is the most commonly used indicator of a patient's level of obesity. For many years, a low BMI was thought to increase the risk of osteoporosis, putting leaner women at a higher risk of sustaining a fracture. It was also thought that a higher BMI afforded a protective effect against sustaining a fracture [4, 5]. This was thought to be a result of Wolff's law, which states that bone in a healthy mammal will adapt to the loads under which it is placed. If loading on a particular bone increases, the bone will remodel over time to become stronger and resist those loads. Or in more simple terms, the heavier an individual is, the stronger their bones will be. Despite this, there is evidence to show that a higher BMI is not in fact protective against sustaining a fracture [6]. This phenomenon has been labelled 'the obesity paradox' [7].

There are multiple studies in the published literature examining the effects of obesity on health. Until relatively recently, there was a paucity of scientific publications looking specifically at the effects of obesity on trauma patients and their management. Most thinking was extrapolated from studies looking at obesity in chronic medical and surgical diseases. The more recent evidence that specifically addresses obesity and trauma is diverse in its origin, and in many cases seems to be contradictory. In this chapter we will attempt to summarise the important aspects of obesity in trauma and its management.

4.2 Basic Concepts

In orthopaedics, the word 'trauma' is usually used to describe a single incident that causes physical harm to the individual involved. The extent of the harm (injury) to the individual is determined by a number of factors, but the primary factor is the level of force that is exerted on the individual. The greater the force applied, the more significant the injury.

The human body is made up of the axial skeleton (skull, spine, ribcage, and pelvis) and the appendicular skeleton (the appendages or limbs). These two different aspects of the skeleton have common and differing roles. The axial skeleton is designed to protect the major organs of the body from harm, including traumatic injuries. The appendicular skeleton is an internal scaffold that is designed to work with the appendicular soft tissues to allow the individual to move around (ambulate).

A fracture is defined as 'a soft tissue injury complicated by the presence of a broken bone'. If the bone is broken, the limb's function may be adversely affected until the break has healed. We often focus on the process of fixing and stabilising broken bones, but in reality the injury to the soft tissues is significantly more important than the injury to the bone(s). Bones generally heal very well once stabilised, but only if the correct environment is maintained by the overlying soft tissues, including the blood supply that brings nutrients to the bone to allow it to heal.

In the event of trauma to the appendicular skeleton, the greater the force applied, the greater the injury to the bone. We know that in the event of direct trauma to a limb, the force that is applied is applied initially to the soft tissues at the point of impact, then through the bone, and then through the soft tissues on the opposite side of the bone. As this energy travels through the limb in this manner, it dissipates as it is absorbed by the tissues that it is passing through, such that the energy on the opposite side from the impact is significantly less than the energy absorbed at the point of impact.

This creates a paradox. Obese patients have, by definition, more soft tissue overlying their bones, and this acts to some extent as protection for the bone. But as we have already stated, the bone is the least important tissue—the soft tissues and their care are what will determine whether the outcome of the injury is good or bad. More soft tissue covering the bone means more soft tissue to be injured. It is important to understand that the absence of a broken bone does not necessarily equate to the absence of a significant injury, especially in obese individuals where their excess adipose tissue has protected the underlying bone, but in doing so has absorbed a significant amount of energy. Obesity has been shown to be associated with an increased mortality after a road traffic accident, even where the injury severity is decreased when compared with non-obese patients [8, 9]. This association demonstrates the 'cushion' effect of obesity protecting the skeleton in road traffic accidents, and the increased mortality is thought to be secondary to other systemic factors. Bloom et al. showed that an elevated BMI was inversely related to chest and abdominal abbreviated injury scores in patients sustaining an abdominal stab wound, and the higher BMI conferred a protective effect against peritoneal violation and the need for operative intervention [10].

4.3 Increased Risk of Falls in Obese Patients

It has been reported that obese individuals are at a greater risk of falling than non-obese individuals [11, 12]. Obese individuals also have a higher incidence of bone fragility, and these two factors combine to result in a higher fracture risk in obese individuals. Obese individuals also have a significantly greater tendency to sustain multiple falls, thereby further increasing their fracture risk [13]. This increased risk of multiple falls can be attributed to a number of factors that are summarised in Table 4.2.

4.3.1 Decreased Physical Activity and Agility

Obese individuals are known to have decreased physical activity levels when compared with non-obese individuals [14]. This lack of physical activity results in reduced muscle strength and poorer agility whilst ambulating because of deconditioning of the muscles and the proprioceptive organs that contribute to balance during physical activity. This decreased agility impairs the obese individual's ability to navigate on uneven surfaces and around obstacles, and impairs their reaction time when a fall occurs, thereby preventing them from protecting themselves from the impact [15, 16].

4.3.2 Postural Instability

It is also known that obesity is associated with postural instability [17]. Postural stability is described as the body's ability to maintain or restore the centre of mass with respect to the base of support, or in simpler terms, to maintain balance relative to your stance and/or gait. Several systems, including the brain, visual, vestibular, and proprioceptive systems, in tandem with the musculoskeletal system, contribute to this control of postural stability whilst standing or walking [18]. Deficits in any of these systems result in postural instability.

4.3.3 Sarcopenic Obesity

Sarcopenic obesity is characterised by a loss of muscle mass due to obesity. Obesity causes a form of low-grade chronic inflammation that results in the release of

Table 4.2 Causes of falls in obese individuals

Decreased physical activity	Lower muscle strength and agility
Reduced agility	Associated with slower reaction time when falling
Postural instability	Decompensated load distribution and gait disturbance
Sarcopenic obesity	Fatty infiltration within muscle and bone
Osteoarthritis	Painful unsteady gait
Comorbidities	Systemic conditions that affect balance and strength

harmful cytokines that are harmful to muscle tissue, resulting in fatty infiltration into muscles that are already weak as a result of decreased activity levels [19]. When sarcopenia is accompanied by osteoporosis, the combined weakness in both muscle and bone is referred to as 'osteosarcopenia' or 'osteosarcopenic obesity syndrome' [19, 20]. This syndrome is thought to be induced primarily by obesity as a form of low chronic inflammation that results in the release of cytokines, which are harmful to bone and muscle tissue [19, 20]. It promotes fatty infiltration of the muscles, decreasing their strength and making them less efficient, thereby increasing the fall risk in the obese patient. Sarcopenic obesity is particularly prevalent in the elderly. The European Working Group on Sarcopenia in Older People (EWGSOP) have shown that the prevalence of sarcopenia increases by 11% in the 50–59 age group and by 37% in those aged 80 or more [21]. It has been shown that older individuals with sarcopenic obesity have a three times greater risk of fracture than those with non-sarcopenic obesity or normal BMI [22]. It has also been demonstrated that older individuals with sarcopenic obesity have a higher incidence of non-vertebral fractures compared with those with sarcopenia or obesity in isolation [22].

4.3.4 Associated Conditions

Obese individuals have an inherent predisposition to osteoarthritis in the weight-bearing joints of the lower limbs [23]. This results from repeated loading of the weight-bearing joints to a level well above that for which they were designed. This can result in advanced osteoarthritis of the hip and knee at a young age in obese individuals. Ankle arthritis is also common in obese individuals, but may be post-traumatic arthritis as certain obese individuals are more susceptible to ankle fractures sustained when falling [24]. Lower limb arthritis of any aetiology is painful and causes the individual to limp and walk with an altered or antalgic gait pattern, thereby increasing their risk of postural instability, falls, and injury [25].

4.4 Bone Fragility

Bone fragility is a condition that is characterised by a deficit in the quantity of the bone present, the quality of that bone, or both [26]. The disease that is characterised by increased bone fragility is called osteoporosis. Osteoporosis is characterised by a decrease in bone mineral density (BMD) and bone mass. This can lead to a decrease in bone strength that increases the risk of fractures in the event of trauma. As stated previously, Wolff's law states that bone in a healthy mammal will adapt to the loads under which it is placed. If loading on a particular bone increase, the bone will remodel over time to become stronger and resist those loads. Or in more simple terms, the heavier an individual is, the stronger their bones will be. In theory.

This logic was previously thought to hold true in humans. It was thought that a lower BMI conferred a greater risk of developing osteoporosis, whilst a higher BMI conferred a degree of protection against fractures [27]. There are a large number of scientific studies that support this theory that an elevated BMI results in a higher BMD, but there is good evidence that this increase in BMD does not confer protection against fractures in obese individuals [6]. The increase in the overall BMD in obese patients is probably not sufficient to compensate for the excess loads placed onto the skeleton, especially during falls onto the upper limbs [28]. This phenomenon has been referred to as 'The Obesity Paradox' [7] and can be attributed to the higher risk of falling in obese individuals, and the increased bone fragility that is associated with adiposity. It also reflects the fact that the relationship between increasing BMI and increasing BMD is not proportionate, with the BMI increasing at a much faster rate than the BMD.

This increased bone fragility can be attributed to a number of inter-related factors, but the entire pathophysiological process is not as yet fully understood [29]. It is a complex process involving multiple organ systems within the body, multiple inter-related inflammatory pathways, and hormonal factors that differ between men and women, and between pre-menopausal and post-menopausal women. The full extent of these interrelated processes is beyond the scope of this chapter. We do know that certain fat-derived hormones (adipokines) are involved in the development of obesity. These adipokines interact with other pro-inflammatory and anti-inflammatory agents that are increased in obesity, resulting in a chronic low-grade inflammatory condition that affects multiple organ systems and increases the risk of complications during orthopaedic and trauma surgery [30]. This low-grade inflammatory condition has been linked with cardiovascular and metabolic complications, infections, and wound- and bone-healing complications.

4.5 Injury Patterns in Obese Patients

It is clear that the risk of fracture is increased in obese individuals. Studies from the United States have shown that adults with a BMI between 25 and 30 have a 15% higher likelihood of being injured after a traumatic event than those with a BMI of less than 25. If they are morbidly obese, their likelihood of injury has been shown to be 48% higher [28, 31, 32]. However, this increased risk of fracture is associated with certain types of fractures, but is not associated with others. This phenomenon is known as 'The Obesity Fracture Site Paradox' as the increased risk of fracture in obese individuals occurs in different anatomical areas to those areas generally associated with osteoporotic fractures [33]. Some studies have shown that the risk of sustaining hip, vertebral, and wrist fractures is lower in obese individuals than would be expected [34, 35]. Conversely, the risk of ankle, upper leg, and humerus fractures has been shown to be higher than average in obese individuals [36, 37]. Other studies have provided evidence that refutes these results, and in some cases directly contradicts them.

There are gender-linked differences in fracture patterns in the obese population too. Caffarelli et al. showed that obese men are at a higher risk of sustaining upper forearm fractures and ankle fractures, but have a lower risk of hip, spine, wrist, forearm, and pelvic fractures [38]. In women, Caffarelli et al. showed similar fracture patterns in obesity, but with an increased incidence of humeral and vertebral fractures [38]. As with many aspects of modern medicine, the outcomes of different studies show different patterns, and the general consensus regarding injury patterns in obese individuals is in a constant state of flux. The Edinburgh group conducted an epidemiological analysis of trauma patients presenting to their hospital over a 1-year period [3]. They showed that in their cohort males showed a positive relationship between obesity and fractures of the proximal humerus, finger phalanges, and the ankle. There was a negative relationship with clavicle and proximal femur fractures. In females, there was a positive relationship with obesity in fractures of the humeral diaphysis, the carpus, and the ankle, and a negative relationship with obesity and fractures of the clavicle, proximal femur, and calcaneus [3].

These anomalous results are thought to be related to the mechanism of falling that occurs in obese individuals. It is hypothesised that the abundance of adipose tissue around the hips and pelvis of obese individuals provides protective padding to these regions in the event of a fall. This hypothesis is supported by the results of the Edinburgh study, where obesity was not associated with proximal femur fractures in either males or females [3]. The legs and upper limbs of obese individuals tend to be less well padded, thereby leaving them at a higher risk of fracture in the event of a fall [39, 40]. It has also been shown that obese individuals are more prone to falling backwards or to the side, rather than the more typical Fall Onto an Out-Stretched Hand (FOOSH) that is associated with wrist fractures [41]. Obese individuals also have a tendency to internally or externally rotate their ankles, thereby theoretically placing them at a higher risk of ankle fractures during a fall [24]. This theory is supported by the Edinburgh study, where both male and female groups demonstrated a positive relationship with obesity and ankle fractures [3].

In higher energy trauma such as road traffic accidents, obese individuals are protected from abdominal and soft-tissue pelvis injuries because of the abundance of adipose tissue in these areas [42]. They are more likely to sustain a pelvic ring injury, however, because the energy absorbed by the abdomen is transferred to the pelvic ring [42]. These patients are also more likely to sustain fractures of the distal femur, ankle, and calcaneus [41–43]. So, obese individuals are at a greater risk of certain specific musculoskeletal injuries, and their mortality rates are higher when subjected to high-energy trauma [28, 31].

Even with lower energy injuries, obese patients show different injury patterns from non-obese patients. Obese patients have a tendency to sustain comminuted fractures, which are often open injuries with greater soft-tissue disruption than non-obese patients [31, 43]. These injuries often occur at the distal ends of long bones. Knee dislocations have also been reported after low-energy injuries in obese individuals, and as with any patient, this injury carries a significant risk of neurovascular injury and the need for amputation [28].

4.6 Practical Considerations: Imaging

Obese patients require special consideration with regards to preoperative and intraoperative radiological assessment. Preoperative trauma radiographs may be more difficult to interpret because of the higher density of soft tissue overlying potential fracture sites. This is particularly relevant at the proximal femur, where it has been shown that obese patients have a higher risk of having an occult ipsilateral fracture of the femoral neck in conjunction with a femoral shaft fracture [28, 44]. This problem is somewhat counterbalanced by the fact that obese patients have a lower incidence of proximal femur fractures because of the protective effect of their abdominal soft-tissue envelope. Where doubt remains, higher level imaging should be performed, most commonly in the form of CT scanning, in order to ensure that proximal femur fractures are not obscured by excessive soft-tissue coverage. This in itself may also pose a problem as the obese patient may be too large to fit into a conventional CT or MRI scanner. Not every centre has direct access to an 'open' scanner, and in an emergency scenario it may not be safe to await transfer to a centre where adequate imaging can be performed. This difficult scenario brings a further dimension to the concept of damage limitation trauma surgery.

Intraoperative imaging may be compromised by body habitus in obese individuals. A standard c-arm may not have a large enough radius of curvature to image a neck or femur fracture in a morbidly obese individual. In these extreme circumstances, the operating table may need to be augmented to accommodate the weight of the patient. Dual tables aligned side-by-side may be required in certain circumstances. With intra-articular fractures, intraoperative arthrography should be considered in patients whereby the joint surface is difficult to visualise as a result of overlying soft tissue [28, 44].

4.7 Practical Considerations: Positioning and Fixation

Non-operative management of appendicular injuries may not be appropriate in obese individuals. This is a particular concern in patients whose obesity and associated medical conditions render them 'high-risk' for surgical intervention, but whose injuries cannot be adequately managed non-operatively. In obese individuals, cast immobilisation of the limbs may be difficult to achieve, and even if a cast can be applied, three-point fixation may not be achievable because of the abundance of soft tissue between the cast and the bone. Even in individuals with central obesity and relatively thin appendages, cast immobilisation may not be appropriate. The classic example of this is the midshaft humerus fracture in an obese individual, where the truncal obesity causes a varus displacement of the humerus at the fracture site [32].

Intra-medullary nailing of femoral fractures poses a series of problems in the obese individual. The standard anterograde nailing of a femoral shaft fracture may be extremely difficult in an obese individual, and retrograde nailing should be considered. It has been shown that retrograde nailing results in less bleeding, less irradiation, and a shorter surgical time in obese patients with femoral fractures [28, 32].

This approach is not appropriate in fractures of the proximal femur or the femoral neck, and an anterograde approach may be necessary. Under these circumstances, the patient should be placed in the lateral decubitus position as this allows easier access to the entry point in the greater trochanter [32]. The largest possible diameter nail should be used, with multiple static locking screws within the construct. These measures increase stability of the fixation and lessen the risk of implant failure or displacement. For reasons already discussed, obese patients are less able to partial-weight-bear, and so the fixation construct must be strong and stable enough to withstand full weight bearing, until the bone has healed sufficiently to support the patient's full weight.

4.8 Complications

Complication rates are higher in obese individuals [42]. The complication risk for pelvic ring fractures is 6.8 times higher in an individual with a BMI greater than 30 than in an individual with a BMI of less than 30. The re-operation rate is 4.7 times higher for an individual with a BMI higher than 30, than an individual whose BMI is less than 30 [42]. Obesity has been shown to be one of the factors that increases the risk of complications and duration of hospital stay in patients with a proximal humerus fracture [45]. Historically, obesity was thought to confer protection against skin and soft-tissue complications in distal tibial fractures, but more recent studies have shown that the opposite is true [42].

Potential perioperative complications include periods of hypoxia, unplanned intubation, increased incidence of pulmonary hypertension, heart failure, and perioperative mortality [46, 47]. Obesity is associated with multiple respiratory abnormalities such as sleep apnoea and hypercapnia, and these patients will have an increased demand for ventilation in the perioperative period [46–48]. Cardiovascular risk factors include atherosclerotic cardiovascular disease, congestive cardiac failure, and cardiac arrhythmias [46–48]. Acute respiratory distress syndrome (ARDS) has been reported to be one of the most common complications experienced by morbidly obese patients, and obese patients have been shown to be twice as likely to develop pulmonary complications following surgery [49, 50].

Also in the postoperative period, obesity has been shown to significantly increase the risk of surgical-site complications in patients undergoing fixation of a femur fracture [51]. This finding is in keeping with similar findings in obese patients undergoing elective arthroplasty or spinal procedures, and has been linked with malnutrition and hypoalbuminaemia [51]. Malnutrition has also been shown to be a significant risk factor for patient morbidity and mortality [52]. Obese patients have a higher mortality risk for both blunt and penetrating trauma compared with non-obese patients. These patients also suffer higher rates of overall complications, specifically in terms of respiratory and infectious complications, deep vein thrombosis, and acute kidney injury [53]. The prevalence of cardiovascular and respiratory complications is 16.6% in the obese trauma patient compared with 5.2% in the non-obese patient [54]. One particular study reports that obese patients have an 82%

increased risk of developing ARDS, a 69% increased risk of cardiac arrest, an 83% increased risk of DVT, a 63% increased risk of unplanned intubation, and are more than twice as likely to develop a pulmonary embolism [54].

References

1. www.nutritioncare.org.
2. Available online: https://www.who.int.
3. Court-Brown CM, Duckworth AD, Ralston S, McQueen MM. The relationship between obesity and fractures. Injury. 2019;50:1423–8.
4. Ravn P, Cizza G, Bjarnason NH, et al. Low Body Mass Index is an important risk factor for low bone mass and increased bone loss in early menopausal women. J Bone Miner Res. 1999;14:1622–7.
5. Asomaning K, Bertone-Johnson ER, Nasca PC, Hooven F, Pekow PS. The association between body mass index and osteoporosis in patients referred for a bone mineral density examination. J Women's Health. 2006;15:1028–34.
6. Sadeghi O, Saneei P, Nasiri M, Larijani B, Esmaillzadeh A. Abdominal obesity and risk of hip fracture. A systematic review and meta-analysis of prospective studies. Adv Nutr. 2017;8:728–38.
7. Fassio A, Idolazzi L, Rossini M, et al. The obesity paradox and osteoporosis. Eat Weight Disord-Stud Anorex Bulim Obes. 2018;23:293–302.
8. Mock CN, Grossman DC, Kaufmann RP, Mack CD, Rivara FP. The relationship between body weight and risk of death and serious injury in motor vehicle crashes. Accid Anal Prev. 2002;45:221–8.
9. Moran SG, McGwin G Jr, Reiff DA, Rue LW 3rd. The association between body habitus, restraint use, and fatality in motor vehicle collisions. Annu Proc Assos Adv Automot Med. 2001;45:107–23.
10. Bloom MB, Ley EJ, Liou DZ, et al. Impact of body mass index on injury in abdominal stab wounds: implications for management. J Surg Res. 2015;197:162–6.
11. Himes CL, Rynolds SL. Effect of obesity on falls, injury, and disability. J Am Geriatr Soc. 2011;60:124–9.
12. Sotiriadi-Vlachous S. Obesity and its relationship with falls, fracture site, and bone mineral density in postmenopausal women. J Frailty Sarcopenia Falls. 2017;2:28.
13. Neri SS, Oliviera JB, Dario AM, Lima R, Tiedemann A. Does obesity increase the risk and severity of falls in people aged 60 years and older? A systematic review and meta-analysis of observational studies. J Gerontol Ser. 2019;75:952–60.
14. Jakicic JM, Davis KK. Obesity and physical activity. Psychiatr Clin North Am. 2011;34:829–40.
15. Vincent HK, Mathews A. Obesity and mobility in advancing age. Mechanisms and interventions to preserve independent mobility. Curr Obes Rep. 2013;2:275–83.
16. Pijnappels M, Maarten BF, vanDieen JH. How early reactions in the support limb contribute to balance recovery after tripping. J Biomech. 2005;38:627–34.
17. Hue O, Simoneau M, Marcotte J. Body weight is a strong predictor of postural stability. Gait Posture. 2007;26:32–8.
18. Loram ID, Lakie M. Direct measurement of human ankle stiffness during quiet standing: the intrinsic mechanical stiffness is insufficient for stability. J Physiol. 2002;545:1041–53.
19. Ilich JZ, Inglis JE, Kelly O, McGee D. Osteosarcopenic obesity is associated with reduced handgrip strength, walking abilities, and balance in postmenopausal women. Osteoporos Int. 2015;26:2587–95.
20. Hirschfeld HP, Kinsella R, Duque G. Osteosarcopenia: where bone, muscle, and fat collide. Osteoporos Int. 2017;28:2781–90.
21. Yazar T, Yazar HO. Prevalence of sarcopenia according to decade. Clin Nutr ESPEN. 2019;29:137–41.

22. Scott D, Seibel M, Cumming R, et al. Sarcopenic obesity and its temporal associations with changes in bone mineral density, incident falls, and fractures in older men. The Concord Health and Ageing in Men Project. J Bone Miner Res. 2017;32:575–83.
23. Reyes C, Leyland K, Peat G, Cooper G, Arden NK, Prieto-Alhambra D. Association between overweight and obesity and risk of clinically diagnosed knee, hip, and hand osteoarthritis: a population based cohort study. Arthritis Rheumatol. 2016;68:1869–75.
24. King CM, Hamilton GA, Cobb M, Carpenter D, Ford LA. Association between ankle fractures and obesity. J Foot Ankle Surg. 2012;51:543–7.
25. Deng Z, Xu J, Long L, et al. Association between hip and knee osteoarthritis with falls: a systematic review and meta-analysis. Int J Clin Pract. 2021;75:e14537.
26. Friedman AW. Important determinants of bone strength: beyond bone mineral density. J Clin Rheumatol. 2006;12:70–7.
27. Asomaning K, Bertone-Johnson ER, Nasca PC, Hooven F, Pekow PS. The association between body mass index and osteoporosis in patients referred for a bone mineral density examination. J Women's Health. 2006;15:1028–34.
28. Sabharwal S, Root MZ. Impact of obesity in orthopaedics. J Bone Joint Surg Am. 2012;94:1045–52.
29. Berry PA, Jones SW, Cicuttini FM, Wluka AE, Maciewicz RA. Temporal relationship between serum adipokines, biomarkers of bone and cartilage turnover, and cartilage volume loss in a population with clinical knee osteoarthritis. Arthritis Rheum. 2011;63:700–7.
30. Conde J, Scotece M, Lopez V, et al. Adipokines: novel players in rheumatic diseases. Discov Med. 2013;15:73–83.
31. Jones CB. Management of upper extremity injuries in obese patients. Orthop Clin North Am. 2011;42:11–9.
32. Streubel PN, Gardner MJ, Ricci WM. Management of femur shaft fractures in obese patients. Orthop Clin North Am. 2011;42:21–35.
33. Rinonapoli G, Pace V, Ruggiero C, et al. Obesity and bone: a complex relationship. Int J Mol Sci. 2021;22(24):13662.
34. De Laet C, Kanis JA, Oden A, et al. Body mass index as a predictor of fracture risk: a meta-analysis. Front Endocrinol. 2005;16:1330–8.
35. Gonnelli S, Caffarelli C, Alessi C, Nuti R. Divergent effects of obesity on fragility fractures. Clin Intero Ageing. 2014;9:1629–36.
36. Prieto-Alhambra D, Premaor MO, Fina Aviles F, et al. The association between fracture and obesity is site dependent: a population-based study in postmenopausal women. J Bone Miner Res. 2012;27:294–300.
37. Bouxsein ML, Szulc P, Munoz F, Thrall E, Delmas PD, Sornay-Rendu E. Contribution of trochanteric soft tissues to fall force estimates the factor of risk, and prediction of hip fracture risk. J Bone Miner Res. 2007;22:825–31.
38. Caffarelli C, Alessi C, Nuti R, Gonnelli S. Divergent effects of obesity on fragility fractures. Clin Interv Aging. 2014;9:1629–36.
39. Gnudi S, Sitta E, Lisi L. Relationship of body mass index with main limb fragility fractures in postmenopausal women. J Bone Miner Metab. 2009;27:479–84.
40. Mignardot JB, Olivier I, Promayon E, Nougier V. Obesity impact on the attentional cost for controlling posture. PLoS One. 2010;5:e14387.
41. Garnero P, Sornay-Rendu E, Clasutrat B, Delmas PD. Biomechanical markers of bone turnover, endogenous hormones and the risk of fractures in postmenopausal women. The OFELY study. J Bone Miner Res. 2000;15:1526–36.
42. Sems SA, Johnson M, Cole PA, Byrd CT, Templeman DC, Minnesota Orthopaedic Trauma Group. Elevated body mass index increases early complications of surgical treatment of pelvic ring injuries. J Orthop Trauma. 2010;24:309–14.
43. Graves ML, Porter SE, Fagan BC, et al. Is obesity protective against wound healing complications in pilon surgery? Soft tissue envelope and pilon fractures in the obese. Orthopaedics. 2010;33 https://doi.org/10.3928/01477447-20100625-27.

44. Modica MJ, Kanal KM, Gunn ML. The obese emergency patient: imaging challenges and solutions. Radiographics. 2011;31:811–23.
45. Neuhaus V, Swellengrebel CH, Bossen JK, Ring D. What are the factors influencing outcome among patients admitted to a hospital with a proximal humeral fracture? Clin Orthop Relat Res. 2013;47:1698–706.
46. Brown CVR, Velmahos GC. The consequences of obesity on trauma, emergency surgery, and surgical critical care. World J Emerg Surg. 2006;1:27.
47. Diaz JJ Jr, Norris PR, Collier BR, et al. Morbid obesity is not a risk factor for mortality in critically ill trauma patients. J Trauma. 2009;66:226–31.
48. Dossett LA, Heffernan D, Lightfoot M, et al. Obesity and pulmonary complications in critically injured adults. Chest. 2008;134:974–80.
49. Ditillo M, Pandit V, Rhee P, et al. Morbid obesity predisposes trauma patients to worse outcomes: a national trauma data bank analysis. J Trauma Acute Care Surg. 2014;76:176–8.
50. Rose DK, Cohen MM, Wigglesworth DF, et al. Critical respiratory events in the postanesthesia care unit: patient, surgical and anesthetic factors. Anesthesiology. 1994;81:410–8.
51. Egbert RC, Bouck TT, Gupte NN, et al. Hypoalbuminemia and obesity in orthopaedic trauma patients: body mass index a significant predictor of surgical site complications. Sci Rep. 1953;2020:10. https://doi.org/10.1038/s41598-020-58987-4.
52. Nelson CI, Elkassabanny NM, Kamath AF, Liu J. Low albumin levels, more than morbid obesity, are associated with complications after TKA. Clin Orthop Rel Res. 2015;473:3163–72.
53. Hatchimonji JS, Kaufman EJ, Vasquez CR, et al. Obesity is associated with mortality and complications after trauma: a state-wide cohort study. J Surg Res. 2020;247:14–20.
54. Bell T, Stokes S, Jenkins PC, Hatcher L, Fecher AM. Prevalence of cardiovascular and respiratory complications following trauma in patients with obesity. Heart Lung. 2017;46:347–50.

5 Obesity and the Upper Limb

Peggy Miller, Bisola Salaja, Ailbhe Kenny, and John T. Cassidy

5.1 Introduction

The relationship between obesity and osteoarthritis of the lower limb is well described in the literature [1]. Less research is available regarding the role of obesity and the upper limb, and the associated risks, complications, and the impact on both surgeon and patient of obesity in this context [2]. In this chapter we endeavour to highlight current knowledge surrounding obesity and total shoulder arthroplasty (TSA) and total elbow arthroplasty (TEA), and questions that remain unanswered in this area.

The upper limb and, in particular, the shoulder and elbow are not weight-bearing joints in the traditional sense. The individual role(s) that mechanical loading and inflammatory reaction in these joints have in generating arthritic change is unclear. The presence of osteophytes, abnormal mechanical stress, and structurally weakened cartilage have all been suggested to cause osteoarthritic pain and changes in the glenohumeral joint [3]. However, the exact mechanism remains unknown. It is most likely a combination of the above that predisposes an obese individual to osteoarthritis. An alteration in mechanical load and abnormal weight-bearing patterns may cause increased joint loading, potentially damaging the articular

P. Miller (✉)
University Hospital Waterford, Waterford, Ireland
e-mail: peggy.miller@nohc.ie

B. Salaja · A. Kenny
National Orthopaedic Hospital Cappagh, Dublin, Ireland
e-mail: bisolasalaja21@rcsi.com; kennyal1@tcd.ie

J. T. Cassidy
University Hospital Limerick, Limerick, Ireland
e-mail: johntcassidy@rcsi.ie

J. M. O´Byrne et al. (eds.), *Musculoskeletal Disease and Obesity*,
https://doi.org/10.1007/978-3-031-63310-2_5

cartilage. In the upper limb, heavier limbs and reduced mobility may also contribute to this [4].

We will examine the demographics of shoulder and elbow arthroplasty patients, potential implications of obesity on surgical goals/functional outcomes, potential intraoperative challenges, complications in this patient cohort, and preoperative patient optimisation before TSA and TEA.

5.2 Demographics of Shoulder/Elbow Arthroplasty Patients

Growing numbers of shoulder and elbow arthroplasty are performed each year across the world. In the United States, annual rates of TSA and TEA doubled from 6% to 13% between 1993 and 2007, and this continues to rise [5]. Similarly, the prevalence of obesity has also increased. It is suggested that by 2030 obesity in the United States will increase from 32% in 2008 to 50–51%, and from 26% to 35–43% in the United Kingdom [6]. Over 625,000 patients required bariatric surgery in the United States between 2015 and 2018 as surgical weight loss treatment [7]. Almost one-quarter of Irish adolescents are living with obesity, and thus, the prevalence of the disease and its associated complications is only set to increase [8]. These population demographics will influence the number of obese patients undergoing TSA and TEA.

The UK National Joint Registry recorded 13,734 total shoulder replacements from 2012 to 2020, with numbers increasing annually from 2012 to 2017. A total of 13,720 elective total shoulder replacements were recorded, with the most frequent indication recorded as osteoarthritis (n = 12,746). Stemmed shoulder replacements were the most common type used for the indication of OA, with 7743 recorded [9]. The Australian Orthopaedic Association Shoulder Arthroplasty Report recorded 27,236 shoulder replacement procedures between 2007 and 2015. This number increased by 70% annually between 2008 and 2014. From this data, the most common indication for TSR was osteoarthritis, with this indication documented for 13,260 or 69.6% of patients [10]. Elective TSR for osteoarthritis was more common in female patients across both registries (68.5% of patients were reported as female in the Australian database and 62.4% in the UK database). The average age was 72.3 and 70 years old in the respective databases. Reverse TSR is used most commonly in both databases, with stemmed remaining more common than unstemmed prostheses.

In the United Kingdom between 2012 and 2020, 2358 total elbow replacements were carried out for elective indications. Inflammatory arthropathy was the most commonly reported indication for elective TER but osteoarthritis was the documented indication for 33.8% of patients (n = 798). Radial head replacement was used more commonly than distal humerus hemiarthroplasty, with 43 radial head replacements being performed for osteoarthritis [9]. Less data for elbow replacement is available for TER use by the AOA but annually 500–600 primary elbow replacements were conducted nationally from 2016 to 2022 [11].

With rates of TSR and TER on the rise and almost 40% of adults globally classified as overweight, more of these surgeries will be performed in this cohort [12]. Inclusion of BMI status is necessary for registries going forward to inform the literature on the rates of TSA and TEA being informed in obese patients.

5.3 Potential Implications of Obesity on Surgical Goals/Functional Outcomes

Obese patients have higher rates of musculoskeletal pain at baseline [13]. Before undergoing TSA, obese patients often report a reduced range of motion at the shoulder joint and also increased pain compared with their counterparts of normal body mass index (BMI) [14]. Reduced range of motion at the glenohumeral joint has also been noted in obese individuals who are asymptomatic for shoulder pain. The proposed causes for this include the inability to internally rotate due to a wider body girth and also a heavier upper limb. Adipose distribution is likely a significant factor in the range of motion at the glenohumeral joint in obese patients [15].

Rotator cuff tendonitis and shoulder pain are associated with elevated BMI and increased waist circumference and waist-to-hip ratio [16]. Scores such as the Short-Form-36 (SF-36) and the Western Ontario McMaster Osteoarthritis Index (WOMAC) for pain are increased in obese patients [13]. With weight loss these pain scores and the prevalence of MSK-related pain have been reduced. Chronic neck and shoulder pain is increased by 20% in obese patients, but exercising for at least 1 h a week is thought to reduce this significantly [17]. Increased rates of upper limb tendinopathies are thought to be due to increased loading on the tendon and metabolic factors, thus contributing to increased pain levels in obese patients [18]. Tendinopathy of the elbow (lateral and medial epicondylitis) is also associated with an elevated BMI. Patients with a BMI >40 are most at risk. These patients are therefore more likely to report chronic pain in the elbow region which can impact occupation-related activities and participation in sport and exercise [19].

Despite these challenges, current research suggests that obese patients can expect improvement in functional outcomes in both aTSA and rTSA [20].

The American Shoulder and Elbow Score, range of motion, the Short-Form-26 Physical Components Survey, and Visual Analog Pain Score were all shown to have improved scores in obese patients post-TSA. Similar functional and symptom improvement postoperatively was reported in obese patients and patients of normal BMI. Increased quality of life (QoL) scores were also shown in obese patients who had undergone surgery [21–23].

Some studies suggest that obese patients can expect a more modest improvement in pain and symptoms compared to other patients post TSA; however, this has not been consistently proven across the literature [20].

While we know that obese patients are at risk globally for musculoskeletal pain in the elbow, for obese patients undergoing elbow arthroplasty preoperative functional scores are yet to be reviewed in the literature.

5.4 Potential Intraoperative Challenges

Increased operating time, blood loss, and pain control are among several challenges identified in obese patients undergoing TSA and TEA. We aim to explore these intraoperative complications and how to mitigate them.

Prolonged surgical time has been reported for shoulder arthroplasty in the obese patient [24]. Jiang et al. reported an increased operative time duration for TSA by increasing BMI categories [25]. Overweight patients took on average 5 min longer than those of normal BMI, obese class 1 were 10 min, and obese class 2 were 13 min longer.

Given that many studies have found that prolonged operative time increases the risk of complications, the apparent correlation between BMI and operative time is concerning [26].

Separately it has been reported that obese patients may lose an increase of 40 mL blood loss [22], thus influencing the rates of postoperative anaemia and the requirement for blood transfusion.

The use of intraoperative tranexamic acid IV has been recommended to reduce blood loss with quick postoperative recovery and earlier patient discharges [27]. While the use of closed suction drains is often used to reduce postoperative blood loss and infection, and to prevent the need for transfusion the contrary has been found for TSA and rTSA [28]. A retrospective review by Erikson et al. found reduced haemoglobin levels in patients who had a drain and longer lengths of hospital stay [29]. This is particularly relevant to obese patients who are more likely to have intraoperative blood loss and longer length of hospital stay at baseline post TSA and rTSA. The role of drains post-elbow arthroplasty is yet to be reviewed in the literature.

The use of irrigation fluids has also been shown to have a detrimental effect on obese patients undergoing shoulder surgery. High irrigation pressure and obesity are risk factors for intraoperative and postoperative airway obstruction. If patients develop high intrathoracic pressure during inspiration and an obstructed airway, they may develop negative pressure pulmonary oedema. Intraoperative airway pressure and neck circumference should be measured intraoperatively to reduce airway-related events, and further research needs to be conducted to establish if obese patients are at risk with the increased use of irrigation fluids [30].

From the anaesthetic perspective, management of the obese patient is more challenging intraoperatively. Obese patients have reduced lung volumes, thus inhibiting their physiological tolerance to surgery. Positive end-expiratory pressure (PEEP) via non-invasive ventilation is recommended to maintain lung recruitment intraoperatively, along with endotracheal intubation [31]. Oral airway resistance and hypercapnia are also reported issues in the intubation of obese patients [32]. Increased chest wall loading further complicates intubation and limited flexion and extension of the neck may inhibit airway insertion.

The intraoperative position of the patient also affects respiratory effort and work of breathing. The beach chair and the lateral decubitus positions are often used in shoulder arthroplasty, along with lateral decubitus or supine positioning in TEA. The beach chair position or reverse Trendelenburg may help reduce intra-abdominal pressure and increase chest wall movement. The lateral position can be associated with a high incidence of airway oedema, and the beach chair has reported incidence of hypotensive or bradycardia episodes—this was reported in rotator cuff repair specifically [30]. Head and trunk elevation may avoid severe oxygen desaturations. The use of preoperative anaesthetic clinics is necessary for these patients and will help mitigate the risk of intraoperative pulmonary complications [31].

Pain management intraoperative can be complicated by obesity. Inter-scalene blocks are commonly used in shoulder surgery. However, their use in obese patients has been associated with increased pulmonary complications. Unplanned admission to ICU has been demonstrated consequence of their use in this population [33]. Diaphragmatic paralysis as associated with these types of blocks increases the incidence of dyspnoea and hypoxic episodes in obese patients [34]. Preoperative anaesthetic clinics are vital in this cohort to predict difficulties, plan for postoperative disposition such as ICU, obtain blood samples in the event of increased bleeding, and plan adequate analgesia management for these patients. General anaesthesia or a combined approach is however associated with higher incidences of hypotension and bradycardia, nausea and vomiting, and analgesia requirements [30].

Careful selection of intraoperative and postoperative analgesia is necessary for the obese patient who is often comorbid. Intravenous opioids and systemic treatments such as non-steroidal anti-inflammatory drugs (NSAIDs) can be useful as proven in rotator cuff repair [30]. Inadequate pain control can lead to increased postoperative complications such as complex regional pain syndrome (CRPS).

Correct dosing of anti-biotic prophylaxis is necessary for reducing intraoperative infection risk. The 2018 International Consensus Meeting on Musculoskeletal Infection has recommended weight-based dosing for cefazolin [27].

5.5 Postoperative Complications for TSA

Postoperatively TSA patients who are classified as obese experienced an increased rate of venous thrombo-embolism, superficial infection, respiratory complications, and longer length of hospital stay [35]. Medical complications are increased in obese patients post-TSA when patients are matched for age, gender, and comorbidities in non-obese patients [24]. This, however, has not been consistently demonstrated across all studies. While research trends may be shown towards increased medical complications post TSA in obese patients, certain researchers report little difference in complication rates between obese and non-obese patients postoperatively [36–39].

Increased rates of revision and mechanical failure have also been reported, but this also remains inconsistent across the literature. In a study by Wagner et al. reviewing over 4456 shoulder arthroplasty cases, they found an increasing BMI was associated with revision, mechanical failure, and superficial infection [40].

An increase in trends showing a prolonged length of stay and a reduced likelihood of direct discharge home has also been identified [41]. Length of stay increased linearly with BMI, with morbidly obese patients staying on average 2.84 days, obese patients staying 2.56 days, and non-obese patients staying 2.52. This study also reported increased rates of postoperative anaemia and respiratory dysfunction which may account for their prolonged hospital stay. Associated costs for patients and health services due to prolonged length of stay need to be reviewed in the Irish Health System.

Increased rates of revision and mechanical failure have also been reported, but this also remains inconsistent across the literature. In a study by Wagner et al. reviewing over 4456 shoulder arthroplasty cases, they found an increasing BMI was associated with revision, mechanical failure, and superficial infection [40].

This has been found in early revision, within 1 year where dislocation was the most commonly cited cause [42]. It has also been demonstrated in longer-term studies of up to 30 years [43]. The proposed cause of these long-term revision rates included the greater production of pro-inflammatory cytokines which can promote synovial inflammation and cartilage degradation.

Despite this TSA is thought to be a safe and effective procedure when done in the obese patient when patients have been reviewed in follow-up clinics for at least 2 years [44].

5.6 Postoperative Complications for TEA

Increased complication rates in TEA compared with THA and TKA are due to the complex anatomy of the elbow joint and the variability of indications for TEA [45].

Obese patients experienced increased rates of venous thromboembolism (VTE) post-TEA and increased infection rates [46]. Increased rates of VTE are common in obese patients and are not specific to TEA. Genetic factors, use of steroids, inflammation, and insulin resistance are thought to contribute to the role of obesity in VTE [47].

Complications of elbow arthroplasty include infection, aseptic loosening, instability, and peri-prosthetic fracture; however, it is unclear if the rates of these complications are increased in the obese patient [48]. The 30-day readmission rate for TEA is similar to that of THA and TKA at 4.4% [49].

Obese patients are also reported to have an increased rate of implant removal post-TEA [50]. Both local and systemic complications are reported to be increased in the obese population at 90-day follow-up post-TEA [51].

Peri-prosthetic infection is comparably higher post-TEA compared with other total joint replacements. The specific reason for this is unknown but younger age at the time of surgery and obesity are increased risk factors for this, and two-stage revision remains the gold-standard treatment for TEA PJI [52]. Infection is the most common cause of unplanned readmissions and re-operations. Certain studies have found patients with a reduced BMI at increased risk relative to obese patients, but this is likely due to the nutritionally deficient state some patients have who have a low BMI. Obese patients are also subject to being malnourished or being nutrient depleted, so it is not possible to say that obesity is a protective factor in readmission and re-operation in TEA [53].

A study by Prior et al. found increased rates of aseptic loosening in obese patients post-TEA. Male sex and opioid use were also found to have an increased predisposition to aseptic loosening [54].

Heterotopic ossification is another known complication that may arise post-TEA. While it may be asymptomatic it can also limit range of motion and lead to poor outcomes. Obesity was not reported to be a risk factor for HO post-TEA but further studies may be required as approximately 1% of patients undergo surgical excision for HO post-TEA [55].

Other studies would suggest that increased risk of complications is not linked to obesity post-TEA but more so with longer operative time. Lack of functional independence and in-patient hospital stay may be associated with increased risk [56].

Revision rates for TEA are described at approximately 14% [57]. When reviewing the 10-year survival rate for TEA revision for mechanical failure has been described as about 88% in non-obese patients compared with 72% in obese patients (BMI >30). Patients with a BMI >40 were found to have a higher risk of revision for all reasons including mechanical failure [58].

In a study of over 700 patients by Baghdadi et al., they reviewed the 10-year survival rate for TEA in the obese patient. They found obese patients to have a rate of mechanical failure at 88% compared with 72% in non-obese. They also found increased rates of extensor mechanism dysfunction and heterotrophic ossification. One-third of the obese patients underwent revision compared with only one-quarter of the non-obese cohort [58].

Diabetic patients who undergo TEA have increased rates of urinary tract infections, pneumonia, cerebrovascular accidents, blood transfusion, and nonroutine discharge. BMI class was not recorded in this cohort, but it may be useful to evaluate if obese patients who have TEA also experience these complications at increased rates [59]. Comorbidities such as COPD and chronic kidney disease have also been shown to complicate in-patient trajectory in patients having TEA and the associated cost of care to the health service [60].

Mortality rates are controversial post-TSA. Some studies have found BMI >30 to be protective in 90-day mortality rates post-TSA [61]. Similar findings for TEA have reported comparable 90-day mortality rates in obese and non-obese patients [58]. These findings are consistent with the well-reported 'Obesity Paradox'.

5.7 Preoperative Considerations

Multidisciplinary team-enhanced recovery programmes have shown improvement in length of stay, functional outcome, and patient satisfaction. Patient education, occupational therapy, and a standardised perioperative regional anaesthetic regimen have all improved patient outcomes post-TSA [62].

A specific Enhanced Recovery Program for elbow arthroplasty is yet to be described. The use of these programmes may help mitigate and plan for some of the complications experienced by obese patients in TSA and TEA.

Careful planning from an anaesthetic perspective is necessary before shoulder arthroplasty as aforementioned. Preoperative planning for the use of a block or general anaesthesia will play a huge role in reducing postoperative pain and the role of postop mobilisation in the TSA and rTSA cohort. Comorbidities such as rheumatoid arthritis will also inform choices [63].

Super-obese is a sub-classification within BMI. It refers to patients with a BMI >50. In a study by Werner et al., super-obese patients were more likely to suffer complications such as infection, loosening, dislocation, revision, and venous thromboembolism [64]. This is different from the data reported for obese patients; however, much of the current literature does not classify patients as obese, morbidly obese, or super-obese. It is unclear at what point this risk increases, and thus, more studies are required to document patient BMI subclass.

Patients who undergo bariatric surgery following TSA have also been reported to have an increased risk of mechanical complications and implant loosening. Rates of mechanical complications and loosening have been found in patients who undergo bariatric surgery following a TSA [65]. The cause of this remains unclear; however, it may be important to consider when patients are being counselled for surgical risk, and it could be prudent to suggest that bariatric surgery take place before TSA if a patient is planned to undergo both procedures.

As we have outlined special considerations need to be made for obese patients undergoing TSA and TEA to reduce risks and improve their postoperative outcomes. Increased complication rates need to be reviewed when selecting surgical candidates and efforts made for preoperative planning and optimisation. When consenting obese patients, risks should be highlighted to patients for informed consent. A multidisciplinary team approach in liaison with anaesthetic colleagues is also necessary to reduce risk. While individual hospitals may have specific postoperative rehabilitation programmes for TSA and TEA, little is available that is specific to the obese patient or a recognised global standard.

Further research is also required on this topic to highlight the number of patients undergoing these surgeries who are obese, the effects of intraoperative positioning specifically in these patients, and the role of enhanced recovery programmes for TSA and TEA.

5.8 Conclusion

Despite the challenges, the current available evidence suggests that patients with a safe procedure can expect improved functional outcomes. Nevertheless, complication rates are higher than those in other cohorts. Careful planning and patient preparation are recommended (as outlined above) in order to mitigate associated risks and facilitate an appropriate consent process. Given the relative paucity of evidence, further research is required to improve the evidence base and improve the care for this increasingly frequent cohort.

References

1. King LK, March L, Anandacoomarasamy A. Obesity & osteoarthritis. Indian J Med Res. 2013;138(2):185–93.
2. Lester JD, Hsu S, Ahmad CS. Occupational hazards facing orthopedic surgeons. Am J Orthop (Belle Mead NJ). 2012;41(3):132–9.
3. Ibounig T, Simons T, Launonen A, Paavola M. Glenohumeral osteoarthritis: an overview of etiology and diagnostics. Scand J Surg. 2021;110(3):441–51.
4. Guilak F. Biomechanical factors in osteoarthritis. Best Pract Res Clin Rheumatol. 2011;25(6):815–23.
5. Day JS, Lau E, Ong KL, Williams GR, Ramsey ML, Kurtz SM. Prevalence and projections of total shoulder and elbow arthroplasty in the United States to 2015. J Shoulder Elb Surg. 2010;19(8):1115–20.
6. Wang YC, McPherson K, Marsh T, Gortmaker SL, Brown M. Health and economic burden of the projected obesity trends in the USA and the UK. Lancet. 2011;378(9793):815–25.
7. Altieri MS, Irish W, Pories WJ, Shah A, DeMaria EJ. Examining the rates of obesity and bariatric surgery in the United States. Obes Surg. 2021;31(11):4754–60.
8. Moore Heslin A, O'Donnell A, Kehoe L, Walton J, Flynn A, Kearney J, et al. Adolescent overweight and obesity in Ireland—trends and sociodemographic associations between 1990 and 2020. Pediatr Obes. 2023;18(2):e12988.
9. Ben-Shlomo Y, Blom A, Boulton C, Brittain R, Clark E, Dawson-Bowling S, et al. Outcomes after joint replacement 2003 to 2020 [Internet]. The National Joint Registry 18th Annual Report 2021 [Internet]. National Joint Registry; 2021 [cited 2023 May 3]. Available from: https://www.ncbi.nlm.nih.gov/books/NBK576849/.
10. Davidson MD, de Steiger PR, Lewis MP, Stoney MJ, Tomkins A, Rainbird DS, et al. Australian Orthopaedic Association National Joint Replacement Registry: annual report. 2018.
11. Elbows [Internet]. AOANJRR. [cited 2023 May 3]. Available from: https://aoanjrr.sahmri.com/elbows.
12. Ritchie H, Roser M. Obesity. Our world in data [Internet]. 2017. [cited 2023 May 8]. Available from: https://ourworldindata.org/obesity.
13. Hooper MM, Stellato TA, Hallowell PT, Seitz BA, Moskowitz RW. Musculoskeletal findings in obese subjects before and after weight loss following bariatric surgery. Int J Obes. 2007;31(1):114–20.
14. Park W, Ramachandran J, Weisman P, Jung ES. Obesity effect on male active joint range of motion. Ergonomics. 2010;53(1):102–8.
15. Allen WE, Lin JJ, Barfield WB, Friedman RJ, Eichinger JK. Shoulder motion decreases as body mass increases in patients with asymptomatic shoulders. JSES Int. 2020;4(3):438–42.
16. Rechardt M, Shiri R, Karppinen J, Jula A, Heliövaara M, Viikari-Juntura E. Lifestyle and metabolic factors in relation to shoulder pain and rotator cuff tendinitis: a population-based study. BMC Musculoskelet Disord. 2010;11(1):165.
17. Nilsen TIL, Holtermann A, Mork PJ. Physical exercise, body mass index, and risk of chronic pain in the low back and neck/shoulders: longitudinal data from the Nord-Trondelag Health Study. Am J Epidemiol. 2011;174(3):267–73.
18. Castro AD, Skare TL, Nassif PA, Sakuma AK, Barros WH. Tendinopahy and obesity. Arq Bras Cir Dig. 2016;29(Suppl 1):107–10.
19. Franceschi F, Papalia R, Paciotti M, Franceschetti E, Di Martino A, Maffulli N, et al. Obesity as a risk factor for tendinopathy: a systematic review. Int J Endocrinol. 2014;2014:670262.

20. Reid JJ, Kunkle BF, Kothandaraman V, Roche C, Eichinger JK, Friedman RJ. Effects of obesity on clinical and functional outcomes following anatomic and reverse total shoulder arthroplasty. J Shoulder Elb Surg. 2022;31(1):17–25.
21. Li X, Williams PN, Nguyen JT, Craig EV, Warren RF, Gulotta LV. Functional outcomes after total shoulder arthroplasty in obese patients. JBJS. 2013;95(21):e160.
22. Pappou I, Virani NA, Clark R, Cottrell BJ, Frankle MA. Outcomes and costs of reverse shoulder arthroplasty in the morbidly obese: a case control study. JBJS. 2014;96(14):1169.
23. Vincent HK, Struk AM, Reed A, Wright TW. Mid-term shoulder functional and quality of life outcomes after shoulder replacement in obese patients. Springerplus. 2016;5(1):1929.
24. Linberg CJ, Sperling JW, Schleck CD, Cofield RH. Shoulder arthroplasty in morbidly obese patients. J Shoulder Elb Surg. 2009;18(6):903–6.
25. Jiang JJ, Somogyi JR, Patel PB, Koh JL, Dirschl DR, Shi LL. Obesity is not associated with increased short-term complications after primary total shoulder arthroplasty. Clin Orthop Relat Res. 2016;474(3):787–95.
26. Cheng H, Clymer JW, Po-Han Chen B, Sadeghirad B, Ferko NC, Cameron CG, et al. Prolonged operative duration is associated with complications: a systematic review and meta-analysis. J Surg Res. 2018;229:134–44.
27. Godlewski M, Knudsen ML, Braman JP, Harrison AK. Perioperative management in reverse total shoulder arthroplasty. Curr Rev Musculoskelet Med. 2021;14(4):282–90.
28. Frye BD, Hannon P, Santoni BG, Nydick JA. Drains are not beneficial in primary shoulder arthroplasty. Orthopedics. 2019;42(1):e29–31.
29. Erickson BJ, Campbell K, Jain A, et al. Are post-operative drains beneficial in total and reverse total shoulder arthroplasty? Orthop Res Traumatol Open J. 2016;1(1):22–7.
30. Maurya I, Garg R, Jain VK, Iyengar KP, Vaishya R. Perioperative anaesthetic considerations for rotator cuff repair surgeries: a current concept review. J Clin Orthop Trauma. 2021;11(17):65–71.
31. Imber DA, Pirrone M, Zhang C, Fisher DF, Kacmarek RM, Berra L. Respiratory management of perioperative obese patients. Respir Care. 2016;61(12):1681–92.
32. Schumann R. Pulmonary physiology of the morbidly obese and the effects of anesthesia. Int Anesthesiol Clin. 2013;51(3):41.
33. Vlessides M. Reconsider interscalene nerve block for shoulder surgery in obese patients [Internet]. Anesthesia Experts. 2019. Available from: https://anesthesiaexperts.com/uncategorized/reconsider-interscalene-nerve-block-shoulder-surgery-obese-patients/.
34. Marty P, Ferré F, Basset B, Marquis C, Bataille B, Chaubard M, et al. Diaphragmatic paralysis in obese patients in arthroscopic shoulder surgery: consequences and causes. J Anesth. 2018;32(3):333–40.
35. Cogan CJ, Flores SE, Freshman RD, Chi HM, Feeley BT. Effect of obesity on short- and long-term complications of shoulder arthroplasty. J Shoulder Elb Surg. 2023;32(2):253–9.
36. Monroe EJ, Hardy R, Holmquist J, Brand JC. Obesity and reverse total shoulder arthroplasty. Curr Rev Musculoskelet Med. 2022;15(3):180–6.
37. Mahmoud S, Dong Y, Loloi J, Gruson KI. Are perioperative complications and clinical outcomes following reverse shoulder arthroplasty adversely affected by obesity? A systematic review. Semin Arthroplasty: JSES. 2021;31(1):147–58.
38. Agarwal AR, Wang KY, Xu AL, Stadecker MJ, Jami M, Miller A, et al. Obesity does not associate with 5-year surgical complications following anatomic total shoulder arthroplasty and reverse total shoulder arthroplasty. J Shoulder Elbow Surg [Internet]. 2022;32(5):947–57. [cited 2023 Feb 8]; Available from: https://www.sciencedirect.com/science/article/pii/S1058274622008242.
39. Garcia GH, Fu MC, Webb ML, Dines DM, Craig EV, Gulotta LV. Effect of metabolic syndrome and obesity on complications after shoulder arthroplasty. Orthopedics. 2016;39(5):309–16.
40. Wagner ER, Houdek MT, Schleck C, Harmsen WS, Sanchez-Sotelo J, Cofield R, et al. Increasing body mass index is associated with worse outcomes after shoulder arthroplasty. J Bone Joint Surg Am. 2017;99(11):929–37.

41. Griffin JW, Novicoff WM, Browne JA, Brockmeier SF. Morbid obesity in total shoulder arthroplasty: risk, outcomes, and cost analysis. J Shoulder Elb Surg. 2014;23(10):1444–8.
42. Werner BC, Burrus MT, Begho I, Gwathmey FW, Brockmeier SF. Early revision within 1 year after shoulder arthroplasty: patient factors and etiology. J Shoulder Elb Surg. 2015;24(12):e323–30.
43. Singh JA, Sperling JW, Cofield RH. Risk factors for revision surgery after humeral head replacement: 1,431 shoulders over 3 decades. J Shoulder Elb Surg. 2012;21(8):1039–44.
44. Statz JM, Wagner ER, Houdek MT, Cofield RH, Sanchez-Sotelo J, Elhassan BT, et al. Outcomes of primary reverse shoulder arthroplasty in patients with morbid obesity. J Shoulder Elb Surg. 2016;25(7):e191–8.
45. Sanchez-Sotelo J. Total elbow arthroplasty. Open Orthop J. 2011;5:115–23.
46. Theodoulou A, Krishnan J, Aromataris E. Risk of complications in patients who are obese following upper limb arthroplasty: a systematic review and meta-analysis. Obes Res Clin Pract. 2020;14(1):9–26.
47. Yang G, De Staercke C, Hooper WC. The effects of obesity on venous thromboembolism: a review. Open J Prev Med. 2012;2(4):499–509.
48. Kwak JM, Koh KH, Jeon IH. Total elbow arthroplasty: clinical outcomes, complications, and revision surgery. Clin Orthop Surg. 2019;11(4):369–79.
49. Zhou H, Orvets ND, Merlin G, Shaw J, Dines JS, Price MD, et al. Total elbow arthroplasty in the United States: evaluation of cost, patient demographics, and complication rates. Orthop Rev (Pavia). 2016;8(1):6113.
50. Griffin JW, Werner BC, Gwathmey FW, Chhabra AB. Obesity is associated with increased postoperative complications after total elbow arthroplasty. J Shoulder Elb Surg. 2015;24(10):1594–601.
51. Werner BC, Rawles RB, Jobe JT, Chhabra AB, Freilich AM. Obesity is associated with increased postoperative complications after operative management of distal humerus fractures. J Shoulder Elb Surg. 2015;24(10):1602–6.
52. Watts A, Duckworth A, Trail I, Rees J, Thomas M, Rangan A. Scoping review: diagnosis and management of periprosthetic joint infection in elbow arthroplasty. Shoulder Elbow. 2019;11(4):282–91.
53. Cutler HS, Collett G, Farahani F, Ahn J, Nakonezny P, Koehler D, et al. Thirty-day readmissions and reoperations after total elbow arthroplasty: a national database study. J Shoulder Elb Surg. 2021;30(2):e41–9.
54. Prior H, Jamil Z, Rodriguez AN, Swiggett SJ, Weisberg MD, Razi AE, et al. Comparison of baseline demographics and risk factors for aseptic loosening following primary total elbow arthroplasty. Eur J Orthop Surg Traumatol. 2023;33(7):3153–8. https://doi.org/10.1007/s00590-023-03550-w.
55. Liu EY, Hildebrand A, Horner NS, Athwal GS, Khan M, Alolabi B. Heterotopic ossification after total elbow arthroplasty: a systematic review. J Shoulder Elb Surg. 2019;28(3):587–95.
56. Colliton E, Clippinger B, Jonczyk MM, Coccoluto N, Cassidy C. Total elbow arthroplasty complications and relation to body mass index: an American College of Surgeons National Surgery Quality Improvement Program database study. Semin Arthroplasty: JSES. 2022;32(3):532–8.
57. Davey MS, Hurley ET, Gaafar M, Molony D, Mullett H, Pauzenberger L. Long-term outcomes of total elbow arthroplasty: a systematic review of studies at 10-year follow-up. J Shoulder Elb Surg. 2021;30(6):1423–30.
58. Baghdadi YMK, Veillette CJH, Malone AA, Morrey BF, Sanchez-Sotelo J. Total elbow arthroplasty in obese patients. J Bone Joint Surg Am. 2014;96(9):e70.
59. Toor AS, Jiang JJ, Shi LL, Koh JL. Comparison of perioperative complications after total elbow arthroplasty in patients with and without diabetes. J Shoulder Elb Surg. 2014;23(11):1599–606.
60. Wickman JR, Chopra A, Goltz DE, Levin JM, Pereira G, Pidgeon T, et al. Influence of medical comorbidity and surgical indication on total elbow arthroplasty cost of care. J Shoulder Elb Surg. 2022;31(9):1884–9.

61. Singh JA, Sperling JW, Cofield RH. Ninety day mortality and its predictors after primary shoulder arthroplasty: an analysis of 4,019 patients from 1976-2008. BMC Musculoskelet Disord. 2011;12(1):231.
62. Morgan ML, Davies-Jones GR, Ibrahim EF, Booker SJ, Bateman M, Tambe AA, et al. Introduction of an enhanced recovery programme for total shoulder arthroplasty: report of a novel pathway. BMJ Open Qual. 2021;10(4):e001371.
63. Beecroft CL, Coventry DM. Anaesthesia for shoulder surgery. CEACCP. 2008;8(6):193–8.
64. Werner BC, Burrus MT, Browne JA, Brockmeier SF. Superobesity (body mass index >50 kg/m2) and complications after total shoulder arthroplasty: an incremental effect of increasing body mass index. J Shoulder Elb Surg. 2015;24(12):1868–75.
65. Cancienne JM, Camp CL, Brockmeier SF, Gulotta LV, Dines DM, Werner BC. Bariatric surgery following total shoulder arthroplasty increases the risk for mechanical complications including instability and prosthetic loosening. HSS J. 2018;14(2):108–13.

Obesity and Spine Surgery

6

Andrew Kelly, Conor McNamee, Hugo C. Temperley, and Stacey Darwish

6.1 Introduction

Mean body mass index (BMI) and the prevalence of obesity among adults in the West continue to rise. The prevalence of obesity in the United States rose to 41.9% during 2017–2020, up from 30.5% between 1999 and 2002. Obesity is defined as a BMI greater than 30 kg/m^2 [1]. This trend is costly in human and economic terms as people with obesity are at an increased risk for multisystem comorbidities including cardiac disease, respiratory illness, diabetes, hypertension, and sepsis. Multiple comorbidities require extensive preoperative optimisation that often involves additional hospital teams, ultimately delaying recovery and causing longer hospital stays. Retrospective analysis revealed obese patients and patients with diabetes had significantly higher hospital charges following anterior cervical decompression and fusion than those with neither of these conditions ($p < 0.05$) [2]. When considering the interplay between low back pain and lumbar disc degeneration, a positive association with obesity has been demonstrated and a dose–response relationship identified [3, 4]. Cross-sectional analysis revealed a positive linear relationship between BMI and overall presence of lumbar disc degeneration on MRI in overweight (OR 1.30 95% 1.03–1.62) and obese (1.79 95%CI 1.17–2.74) subjects [3]. Data from the

A. Kelly (✉) · C. McNamee
National Spine Injuries Unit, Mater Misericordiae University Hospital, Dublin, Ireland

UCD School of Medicine, Dublin, Ireland
e-mail: andrew.kelly3@health.wa.gov.au; conor.mcnamee@ucdconnect.ie

H. C. Temperley
Department of Surgery, Trinity Centre for Health Sciences, St. James's Hospital and Trinity College Dublin, Dublin, Ireland
e-mail: temperlh@tcd.ie

S. Darwish
National Spine Injuries Unit, Mater Misericordiae University Hospital, Dublin, Ireland

J. M. O´Byrne et al. (eds.), *Musculoskeletal Disease and Obesity*,
https://doi.org/10.1007/978-3-031-63310-2_6

Osteoarthritis Initiative, a multicentre prospective study involving 4796 participants, showed that 47.4% of patients with normal or underweight BMI complained of low back pain compared with 72.8% patients of morbidly obese [4]. The mechanism by which obesity causes lumbar disc degeneration is contentious and may be due to increased loading forces, inflammatory mediators, vascular insufficiency [5], or genetic effects [6].

The numbers requiring spinal surgery that meet the criteria of overweight or obese are alarming. Retrospective analysis involving all 24,196 patients who underwent lumbar surgery in the United States from 2006 to 2011 showed the overwhelming majority (79.3%) to be overweight or obese [1]. Marquez-Lara et al. also reported this cohort was associated with technically more difficult procedures, longer operating times, surgical-site infections, and venous thromboembolism [1, 10, 11]. Technical challenges of spinal surgery in the obese patient include, but are not limited to, obstruction of the surgical field and greater required microdissection, positioning challenges, higher estimated blood loss, and longer operative times. Furthermore, obese patients provide additional anaesthetic challenges. Airway complications, metabolism of anaesthetic agents in adipose tissue, and higher likelihood for HDU admission following surgery are repeatedly mentioned in anaesthetic literature in relation to obese patients [7–9]. Nevertheless, a significant proportion of obese patients presenting with spinal pathology require surgical intervention, and despite inherent concerns, can achieve similar outcomes to non-obese cohorts through tailored treatment strategies and optimisation of perioperative management [10, 11]. Advancements in novel surgical strategies, including minimally invasive surgery, computer navigation, and robotics, could make spinal surgery in obese patients more feasible and help reduce surgical complications [12–22]. The purpose of this narrative review is to summarise the implications of obesity on the spine patient's clinical pathway, as well as strategies to optimise patient care.

6.2 BMI and the Degenerative Spine

Obesity has been linked with degenerative lumbar pathology, including spondylolisthesis [23], stenosis [24], and intervertebral disc herniation [25]. The exact etiopathogenesis of this interaction has not yet been rigorously defined; however, traditionally it has been said that excessive, repeated axial loading overwhelms reparative mechanisms over time [25]. This is presumed to occur, in part, because the disc is avascular and therefore perfused via diffusion, affording it only a limited capacity for regeneration and a propensity towards ischaemia in those with atherosclerosis. This theory is challenged by the link between obesity and osteoarthritis in non-weight-bearing areas such as the hands [26, 27]. This suggests a mechanism of cartilage degradation which extends beyond excessive force across the joint, instead favouring some obesity-specific metabolic process. Obesity is a well-recognised proinflammatory state wherein adipocytes exert endocrine influence via release of adipokines, most notably Leptin [28], whose receptors are found on the disc and have been linked with its degeneration in vitro [29]. Leptin is thought to be the primary metabolic link between obesity and osteoarthritis [30, 31] due to its deleterious effect on collagen. Mediators released in the metabolic syndrome have been shown to hypertrophy the spinal ligaments [24] and cumulative spondylotic changes can narrow the vertebral canal. The degenerative process may be affected by numerous weak-to-moderate genetic influences. Those genes with the highest level of evidence when reviewed tend to be those which are biologically plausible, such as variations in type XI collagen [32]. The exact process which links obesity and degeneration of the spine is likely multifactorial. Until a robust etiopathogenesis is elucidated through preventative or early interventional studies, the surgeon must focus on patient optimisation.

6.3 Conservative Management

Obese patients are more challenging surgical prospects for a multitude of reasons. A myriad of serious health conditions, including atherosclerosis, obstructive sleep apnoea, hypertension, and diabetes [33], make the avoidance of surgery, where possible, seem a reasonable venture in obese patients with spinal pathology. In saying this, conservative management strategies should be thoroughly explored before considering surgical intervention.

The North American Spine Society recommends, in the absence of red flag symptoms, conservative therapies be used first line for people presenting with lumbar back pain with or without radiculopathy [34]. The long-term efficacy of conservative measures for lumbar disc herniation is contested, although stabilisation exercises may be beneficial compared to no intervention [35]. Many tested exercise regimes have less than 50% patient compliance [36]. Obese patients with degenerative spondylolisthesis and disc herniation have been shown to derive less benefit from non-operative treatments than non-obese patients [37]. Sub-analysis of the Spine Patient Outcomes Research Trial (SPORT) found that obese patients with degenerative spondylolisthesis (DS) treated conservatively had SF-36 physical function scores that worsened from baseline by a mean of 3.5 compared with a mean improvement of 13.9 from baseline in non-obese patients in the same time period ($p < 0.0001$) [38].

Transforaminal epidural steroid injections provide modest but immediate pain relief and improved function in radiculopathies [39]. Preliminary evidence implies this holds true when used for obese patients [40]. When comparing overweight and obese groups to normal-weight patients, no significant differences were found in percentage improvement in pain following TESI ($p = 0.07154$, $p = 0.4566$) [40]. A 2022 retrospective investigation of 343 participants has shown no significant change in mean Oswestry Disability Index (ODI) score at 3 months post-TESI in the non-obese versus obese patient group (−5.74 vs. −7.33, $p = 0.46$) [41]. The benefits of steroid injections are, however, fleeting, often necessitating repeat treatments and there is no effect on long-term rate of escalation to surgery [42]. In the general cohort, lumbar epidural steroid injections (LESI) guided via palpation of landmarks are prone to interpretation error [39]. One can reasonably expect this issue to be more pronounced in obese patients. Evidence shows that when using a fluoroscopic guidance, procedure time is significantly greater for obese patients [43]. In this study, the interlaminar approach took less time at all BMIs than the transforaminal route. The authors attribute this in part to loss of resistance techniques which may reduce the practitioner's reliance on imaging during interlaminar LESI. The time difference was also largest at the L5/S1 level, and post hoc analysis revealed a greater proportion of long needles used for this area. The deterministic and stochastic consequences of this radiation exposure are beholden to the radio-sensitivity of the involved tissues and the total effective dose received. These values are difficult to calculate and subject to significant error [44]; as such, the clinical significance of fluoroscopy time in obese patients is uncertain.

Epidural lipomatosis (EL) is a pathological overgrowth of adipose tissue in the epidural space and may lead to compressive symptoms [45]. Prevalence has been estimated at 2.5% among those receiving dedicated spine MRI [46]. The population used to make this approximation had an average BMI of 28. The likelihood of development of EL scales linearly between BMIs of 28–35 (Spearman coefficient 0.73, $p < 0.01$) [47] and there is an established link with steroid exposure [48]. Numerous case reports note its development after LESI [47, 49–51], and cross-sectional investigation yields an odds ratio of 3.48 among patients exposed to epidural injections [46]. Risk appears to scale with the number of steroid injections received, approaching almost 100% prevalence among patients with four or more treatments in one case series [47]. In this study the lesions were found to be predominantly located in the L5/S1 area.

6.4 Preoperative Optimisation

6.4.1 Preoperative Medical Evaluation

Obese patients often possess a variety of comorbidities. Thorough preoperative evaluation is fundamental before considering spine surgery in this patient group. With regards to cardiovascular conditions linked with obesity, hypertension and atherosclerosis are significant when considering increased physiological stress response to surgery and the associated risk of myocardial infarction. Obesity increases the risk of arrythmias, likely due to fatty and ischaemic remodelling of the myocardium. Arrythmias predispose patients to embolic events leading to CVAs and downstream occlusion. Respiratory issues are related to reduced lung compliance and decreased functional residual capacity. Obstructive sleep apnoea and obesity hyperventilation syndrome are well-recognised phenomena in obesity. Other common obesity-related illnesses include non-alcohol fatty liver disease and metabolic conditions, including diabetes, hyperlipemia, and thyroid dysfunction. This is a complex list of comorbidities which should be handled at a preoperative anaesthetic clinic well in advance of the proposed surgery. Preoperative evaluation should include routine blood tests; full blood count, electrolytes, liver function tests, lipids, HbA1c, thyroid function tests, and coagulation profile. Additional tests should include echocardiogram (ECG), chest radiographs, and pulmonary function tests, If any abnormalities are noted, further diagnostics may be needed such as cardiac stress testing, echocardiogram, or referral to specialist clinics for disease evaluation and optimisation.

6.4.2 Preoperative Weight Loss

Preoperative weight loss (WL) may form part of conservative therapy for obese patients. This approach is well researched in those due for bariatric surgery. In such a context, it is likely this practice reduces postoperative complications such as infection [52]. Patients undergoing operations for degenerative spinal disease show better performance outcomes following a 2-month protocol, including regular exercise, pain management, and protein supplementation prior to surgery [53]. Non-surgical WL produces improvements in pain scores and Oswestry Disability Index score for low back pain and disability [54]. Diet and exercise programs are, however, limited as participants generally lose weight for 6 months and regain it steadily thereafter [55]. In other disciplines, diet, exercise, and education are successfully used as a form of prehabilitation for surgery, but at present there is only low-quality, conflicting evidence for this practice in spine operations [56]. Currently, there is a paucity of evidence regarding enhanced recovery after surgery (ERAS) evidence-based protocols in spine surgery. The ERAS society working group recently published recommendations for perioperative care in lumbar fusion detailing 22 ERAS items for consideration in lumbar fusion [57]. Weight loss or weight optimisation, however, does not feature in this list.

Bariatric surgery (BS) produces greater and more durable WL than non-operative interventions [58], with the average patient achieving between 30 and 60 kg of WL [59]. The American Society for Metabolic and Bariatric Surgery guidelines recommend a BMI of 35–40 without comorbidities or 30–35 with significant comorbidities as an indication for BS [60]. BS alone can produce significant and quantifiable reductions in back pain [61] and has been associated with clinical resolution of spine pathology [62]. This investigation involving 4351 bariatric surgery patients looked at the number of days post-surgery until spinal diagnoses were no longer documented in patient records, termed by the authors as 'loss of diagnosis' (LOD). LOD was as follows for the following lumbar pathologies; lumbar stenosis (90 d: 48%, 720 d: 91%), lumbar disk herniation (90 d: 61%, 720 d: 93%), and lumbar spondylolisthesis (90 d: 37%, 720 d: 87%) ($p < 0.05$). Cervical symptomatology showed similar trends of improvement post BS, with comparable LOD rates at 90 d when comparing cervical vs. lumbar degeneration ($p = 0.058$) [62].

Furthermore, BS prior to spinal surgery has been shown to reduce the rates of device-related complications, DVT, and haematoma [63, 64]. Recent evidence suggests BS confers a significantly reduced risk of postop complications in elective anterior cervical discectomy and fusions (ACDF) [65]. A total of 6128 ACDF patients with a BMI > 35 were followed for 90 days. Of these, 411 had received BS within 2 years prior to ACDF. Those with a history of BS showed a significantly reduced rate of 90-day pulmonary complications (6.6% vs. 12.7%, OR 0.53, $p = 0.002$), cardiac complications (15.3% vs. 24.2%, OR 0.69, $p = 0.012$), sepsis (9.5% vs. 15.1% OR 0.69, $p = 0.035$), and 90-day readmissions (3.9% vs. 8% OR 0.53, $p = 0.015$). BS prior to adjacent operations such as total hip arthroplasty (THA) and total knee arthroplasty (TKA) may also be advantageous [66]. Data collected between 1997 and 2011 from a State-wide New York Database shows that the risks for in-hospital complications were lower for THA and TKA performed after BS (OR 0.25, $p < 0.001$ and OR 0.69, $p = 0.021$). One study found that spine surgery patients with a history of BS had higher rates of dysphagia, shock, and acute respiratory distress syndrome (ARDS) than obese patients without prior BS [63]. However, this study also found that the overall complication rate was lower among spine surgery patients with a history of BS (38.8% vs. 55.4%, $p < 0.001$).

Conversely, BS is not without its disadvantages. Preliminary studies have shown that bone mass is reduced after BS, particularly at the hip, with authors hypothesising this is related to skeletal unloading [67]. Secondary hyperparathyroidism is common after BS, especially gastric bypass procedures, on account of malabsorption of vitamin D as the functional length of the small intestine is shortened [68]. A recent meta-analysis suggests global fracture risk is increased after BS [69]. The risk for any fracture type was higher in the BS group compared to the non-BS group (RR 1.29, 95%CI = 1.18–1.42). Increased fracture risk was most pronounced in the appendicular regions (RR 1.42 95%CI 1.08–1.87) and lesser in the axial skeleton. This may be because cortical bone loss predominates in postoperative hyperparathyroidism [67] while the vertebral column, which is largely composed of trabecular bone, is relatively spared from the action of PTH from a densitometric, although not microarchitectural, perspective [70]. These mechanisms are, however, contested as there is significant evidence to suggest the catabolic process is mediated through gut-derived and obesity-related hormones [71].

6.4.3 Imaging

Plain radiographs are often still the first diagnostic test ordered in traumatic, malignant, or degenerative spine presentations due to low cost and ease of acquisition [67]. This modality is relatively insensitive compared to advanced imaging and is further limited in obese patients due to reduced penetration, increased scatter [68], longer exposure time, and greater motion artefacts [69].

MRI has become a necessary prerequisite in caring for spine patients in recent years due to the proliferation of pathological findings which are used for prognostication and operative planning [67]. Most MRI machines have industry standard weight limits of 160 kg and a maximal patient diameter of 60 cm [70]. Typically the quoted maximum diameter is true only in the horizontal plane as in the vertical plane 15 cm must be subtracted to account for the table thickness [70]. Patients unable to avail of conventional MRI can be referred for 'open MRI' which has a larger aperture but produces lower quality images; however, these are still generally of diagnostic quality [68]. CT is beset with similar physical pitfalls as MRI in the obese cohort [69] with image quality degraded due to excessive adipose tissue. Even myelogram may be limited in the obese patient group. Suboptimal preoperative imaging can lead to poor surgical planning and inappropriate intervention.

Intraoperatively imaging difficulties compromise surgeon accuracy in obese patients. Pedicle screw insertion is challenging, and the rate of misplacement when using fluoroscopy is highly variable [71, 72]. A retrospective enquiry has associated obesity with pedicle wall penetration, with the authors suggesting that this is in part due to blurred intraoperative imaging [73]. Fluoroscopic imaging systems are designed to compensate for increased adiposity by increasing their output; however, when used at maximum settings, image quality becomes compromised [73].

6.5 Anaesthesia

Anaesthetic issues are commonplace in all surgeries involving obese patients [79]. Tracheal intubation is more difficult for anaesthesiologists to perform in obese patients [80]. Narrow airways are common in patients with obstructive sleep apnoea. Fibreoptic intubation may be a necessary technique to overcome such difficulty.

Airway management remains a challenge in all obese patients because their safe apnoea period (SAP), time period before oxyhaemoglobin (Sp02) drops to dangerous levels, is relatively shorter in the obese patient [74]. Recent advances in oxygenation techniques involving 'diffusion' oxygenation may help increase SAP [75]. One such development is trans-nasal humidified rapid insufflation ventilatory exchange (THRIVE) which combines the benefits of apnoeic oxygenation with continuous positive airway pressure (CPAP) [75].

Obesity has significant effects on the metabolism and pharmacokinetics of most anaesthetic agents, including propofol, the most commonly used drug for the induction of anaesthesia [76]. Propofol is often used for total intravenous anaesthesia (TIVA) during spine procedures as the volatile gases ordinarily used for maintenance interfere with intraoperative neurological monitoring [77].

Weighing the obese patient to accurately titrate propofol can be logistically difficult, and in this group further calculations must be performed to obtain an adjusted body to avoid overdosing [78]. The majority of spine surgeries involve prone positioning. Prone positioning carries with it added airway challenges and reduces cardiac index by 12–24% compared to supine positioning [79].

6.6 Perioperative Considerations

6.6.1 Thermoregulation

Intraoperative hypothermia commonly occurs during spine procedures, irrespective of BMI [76], because all general anaesthetics incur a profound reduction in core body temperature [74]. In obese patients, thick subcutaneous tissue necessitates additional retraction and lengthens operating time [37]. Long surgery is a risk for hypothermia; however, obesity itself is protective [75]. In a prospective study of patients undergoing mixed surgical procedures, those with BMI > 40 and BMI < 30 experienced similar temperature reductions as the operations progressed [77]. Hypothermia slows haemostasis, impairs wound healing, is linked with wound infections, and can delay emergence from anaethesia [78]. Even a mild core body temperature decrease of 2 °C can lengthen post-anaesthetic recovery by 40 min [79]. Forced air warming blankets have been used during spine surgery to prevent this [80] and are well researched in other specialities [81]. These devices can be impractical for the very obese having up to 30% rate of failure when used for patients with BMI > 40 due to tearing, impaired expansion, or excessive heat production [77]. Alternative strategies to prevent hypothermia include preoperative warming, patient insulation, and warmed fluid administration [81]. These may have a greater role to play in the obese patient.

6.6.2 Position

Obese patients require a larger degree of surgical exposure and soft-tissue dissection to access the spine, resulting in more intraoperative blood loss [82]. A meta-analysis suggests a greater mean difference in blood loss in spine surgery involving obese patients (MD = 28.89, 95%CI 14.86–45.65) [82]. Prone positioning of obese patients markedly increases intraabdominal pressure, further exacerbating epidural bleeding [83]. Even when minor, bleeding can obscure the operative field. Prone positioning has also been linked to higher incidences of peripheral neuropathies, compartment syndrome, and pressure ulcers in obese patients [84]. Lengthy surgeries in obese patients have been linked with vision loss due to a prolonged period of increased intraocular pressure during procedures [85]. Stretch injuries to the brachial plexus have been reported; thus, it is important to keep shoulder abduction less than 90 degrees and all bony prominences should be carefully padded. Closed frame tables, such as a Wilson frame, may contribute to increased intrabdominal pressure, leading ultimately to decreased venous return. In mitigation, various frames have been developed which allow the abdomen to hang more freely while the patient is prone, so-called open-frame tables. The first of these was designed in 1969 by Relton and Hall in which two parallel but separate V-shaped supports were devised to provide stability for deformity corrective procedures. The downside to the abdomen hanging freely is the protentional for hyperextension of the vertebral column which may be intensified by the mass effect of the obese abdomen. Bariatric straps may be used to support the freely hanging abdomen. In addition, supporting the abdomen and offloading the load on the patient's spine, these straps allow for free passage of intraoperative imaging devices such as the C-arm around the operating table. The Jackson spinal table (Mizuho Osi, CA) is an alternative open-frame design and has a weight capacity of 227 kg. Horizontal bolsters may alternatively be used. A recent prospective study found horizontal bolsters (H) superior to a conventional Wilson frame (W), resulting in lower intra-abdominal pressure (IAP) and lesser bleeding during lumbar laminectomy and fusion in obese patients [86, 87].

IAP at 10 min in the W group was significantly higher at 11.44 ± 1.61 mmHg compared to 9.56 ± 1.92 mmHg in group H ($p = 0.001$). Mean blood loss was reported to be 440.40 ± 176.98 ml in group W versus 317.20 ± 91.04 ml in group H ($P = 0.0003$).

6.6.3 Nonelective Surgery

Trauma precludes the ability to optimise the preoperative period for surgery and adds the challenge of the need for timely intervention. From first response to post-operative recovery, it can be expected for all stages of trauma management in obese patients to be met with time-expending complications unless trauma centres are adequately prepared. The initial stabilisation of unstable spinal fractures can require customised braces, vests, and cervical collars in obese patients. Establishing peripheral intravenous access and monitoring vital signs is often difficult in obese patients, meaning invasive monitoring and central access lines are often required earlier in the management of these patients. Establishing a definitive airway is a well-recognised anaesthetic challenge in obese patients owing to anatomical and physiological features. Increased neck circumference, reduced lung volumes, and reduced chest wall compliances are the problems commonly cited. The inability to hyperextend the neck due to associated spinal cord injuries adds to the difficulty of establishing an airway. Once the patient is stabilised, the challenge of patient transfer then comes into focus. Traditional stretchers have average size limitations of 270–318 kg. The need for specially designed ambulances and helicopters is often needed to transfer morbidly obese patients with small emergency helicopters reporting maximum carrier weight of 135 kg. Transferring an obese patient from a trauma scene necessitates special equipment and expertise, which is often not available in remote areas. Once arriving at a trauma centre, obese patients will face imaging constraints. MRI is the gold standard for assessing spinal trauma where there is a concern for cord injury, but due to obese patients' dimensions, compromised preoperative imaging is achieved through CT, with image quality often degraded due to excess soft-tissue overlying bony anatomy. Inadequate preoperative imaging can lead to incorrect diagnoses and increased surgical risk. A 2013 case series from an Australian trauma centre composed of six morbidly obese patients involved in spine trauma reported preoperative delays in transfer and barriers to imaging. Intraoperatively, the authors reported positioning challenges, longer operative times, instrument constraints, and even wrong-level surgery. Following surgery difficulties included nursing issues, delayed mobilisation, DVTs, and PEs [86, 87]. Treatment challenges around obese patients extend to all areas of trauma. Obese patients have worse outcomes when involved in trauma, resulting in ICU admission. A prospective study over a 2-year period involving 1167 trauma patients admitted to the ICU had a twofold increased risk of infection and 7.1 times greater mortality than non-obese patients (95% CI 2.06–8.9) [88, 89]. The authors cite prolonged requirements for ventilation and indwelling devices such as central line and Foley catheters as potential reasons for poorer outcomes in obese patients. Delays in intervention in spine trauma have particular implications on neurological outcomes. Greater resourcing of emergency response units and trauma centres, with a focus on spinal trauma in obesity, is fundamental to offsetting the burden of a growing obese population.

6.6.4 Advanced Surgical Techniques

Minimally invasive surgical (MIS) approaches have gained acceptance in many disciplines and are increasingly popular among spine surgeons [88, 89]. Endoscopic lumbar discectomy is an innovative alternative to traditional open microdiscectomy (OD). This may be performed via the transforaminal (TELD) or intralaminar (IELD) window. A meta-analysis suggests percutaneous endoscopic lumbar discectomy (PELD) yields equivalent functional outcomes as OD without an increase in complication rate [12]. In this investigation, the length of stay was reduced among patients who received PELD (weighted mean difference = −3.30 d [−5.30 to −1.29]), suggesting that this technique is suitable for day cases and allows for a faster recovery period which may help avoid some of the postoperative complications seen in prolonged admission courses involving obese patients. IELD has been developed for use in those who are unsuitable for PELD due to a high iliac crest or conjoined nerve route [13]. Both options boast significantly reduced soft-tissue damage; however, spine surgeons are not trained to do these as standard and the learning curve may be steep [14].

Minimally invasive transforaminal lumbar interbody fusion (MISTLIF) is a posterior approach spinal fusion that minimises iatrogenic soft-tissue and muscle injury [90]. According to a meta-analysis, these effects confer significantly less blood loss and a shorter length of stay (LOS) versus traditional open TLIF in the general cohort [90]. Blood loss was of 247.82 ml in MIS TLIF vs. 568.18 ml in open TLIF ($P < 0.00001$). Mean LOS was found to be 5.05 d in MIS TLIF vs. 6.92 d in open TLIF ($P < 0.00001$). A meta-analysis by Tan et al. echoes these findings of reduced blood loss and shorter hospital stays, with the addition of MITLIF causing 3.8 times fewer dural tears than open TLIF (95%CI 1.61–9.87, $P = 0.003$) [91]. The authors propose that improved lighting and magnification during minimally invasive procedures allows better visualisation of the dura. Of note, MIS appears to reduce the risk of SSI [92, 93] which is elevated at baseline in obese patients. A large retrospective study calculates an almost sevenfold reduction in SSI when minimally invasive techniques are used in place of open procedures for lumbar decompression and/or fusion for degenerative disease (0.5% vs. 3.3%, $P = 0.0003$) [92].

Computer navigation (CN) is growing in relevance as MIS gains popularity and the visual field becomes ever smaller. Since the C-arm, a mobile fluoroscopic imaging tool, was developed in 1955, medical engineers have looked to bridge the gap between preoperative imaging and intraoperative planning. Historically surgeons would rely less on anatomic landmarks alone, prior to the advent of intraoperative imaging. With the evolution of cross-sectional images from X-rays, first described by Godfrey Hounsfield in 1971, intraoperative imaging has been able to rapidly progress. The concept of 'computer-assisted surgery' was coined by Brown, Roberts, and Wells in 1983 when CT images were integrated with neurosurgical interventions. Four years later the first stereotactic and spinal biopsies were performed under CT guidance. Sustained advances in engineering led to the development of the O-arm (Medtronic, Dublin) in 2005 [94]. This three-dimensional CT imaging system allows for a 360-degree scanning. The technology has paved the way for navigated spinal surgery as, relative to fluoroscopy, it provides higher quality images, with a larger field of view. The CT images produced by the newer generation systems (O-arm II) allow for continuous stacking of multilevel spinal images and remove the need for a pause in surgery. Pedicle screw placement is the most common application of computer navigation to date. Multicentre research in percutaneous lumbar screw placement [17] confirms reduced average fluoroscopy usage per pedicle in CN compared to traditional fluoroscopy-guided placement (6.6 s vs. 9.6 s $P < 0.001$). The CN group also experienced less than half of the breach rate of the control group (3% vs. 7.2% $P = 0.055$). Newer intraoperative CT scanners have since been developed, including Airo and SpineMask Tracker, which reportedly produce less scatter radiation and better image quality whilst addressing errors in stereotaxis compared to the original O arm.

Robotic surgical systems are the latest integration of MIS and CN. The first human robotic-assisted surgery was performed in 1985 using PUMA 200, a robotic arm, to place a biopsy cannula. The robotic arm evolved into the well-known Da Vinci Surgical system which is commonly being used today for renal, cardiac, and gynaecological surgeries, The first spinal surgical robot, SpineAssist (Mazor Robotics Ltd), was introduced in 2004 and later followed by Renaissance in 2011. Their designs have successfully been used alongside percutaneous approaches to help increase the accuracy of screw placement and mitigate risk [15, 18]. Robotic Navigation (RN) allows surgeons to place larger screws with greater fixation strength compared to skin-based intraoperative navigation [15]. Newer generation RN systems, including the Mazor X (Mazor Robotic Ltd), allow for more real-time intraoperative planning with more accurate skin incision, screw length, and screw positioning. Comparison studies using new-generation RN have shown positioning accuracy levels greater than 99% in the robotic study group versus 92–95% in the CT-navigation cohort [19–22]. RN may also decrease radiation exposure resulting from fluoroscopic guidance in MIS. An average radiation exposure time of 34 s per screw for robotic-assisted insertion versus a mean of 77 s for conventional has been reported [19, 21]. Despite its potential for improved accuracy, the high initial cost, and technical challenges, the need for further training has slowed the rollout of RN systems in spine surgery. Early retrospective investigations of obesity and robotic navigation suggest that a BMI > 30 portends screw misplacement with an OR of 2.5 [16, 20, 22]. This may occur due to distortion of the guidewire by increased pressure from soft tissue and subsequent alteration in the trajectory of screws [16]. It seems likely that as these technologies become more widely available and surgeon skill improves, failure rate will decrease. Surgeons can be reasonably expected to feel hesitant to use novel technologies for these high-risk patients during early adoption.

The combination of robotic and navigation systems is an important step in closing the gap between surgical planning and execution.

6.7 Postoperative Period

There is a complex relationship between postoperative complications following spine surgery and obesity [10, 33]. Slower mobilisation, a greater frequency of venous thromboembolism (VTE), and higher reoperation rates with variable long-term functional outcomes have been cited as postoperative concerns in obese patients undergoing spine surgery [38, 82, 95].

6.7.1 Complication Rates and Mobilisation

Obese patients are often less mobile at baseline and encounter more difficulty in mobilising postoperatively for a variety of reasons. Mobilisation may be delayed due to difficult pain management because of greater soft-tissue dissection and increased effective dosing requirements of lipophilic opioids. Greater trauma may also require drains to remain in place for longer, causing further infection risk and delays in recovery. Obese patients are more likely to experience incidental durotomy than non-obese patients (OR = 1.34, $P < 0.0001$) [96]. This common complication may directly postpone mobilisation due to pain, neurological deficits, or infection and because bedrest is commonly prescribed to aid healing. The negative correlation between patient mobilisation time and postoperative complications such as pressure sores and respiratory complications is well established [95]. In a retrospective investigation of 420 patients with incidental durotomy [97], those resting >24 h experienced increased wound complications (8.66% vs. 15.89%, $p = 0.043$) and increased length of stay (7.24 ± 4.23 d vs. 4.47 ± 3.64 d, $p < 0.0001$) compared to those resting <24 h. One may expect these differences to grow in tandem with BMI.

Obese patients, particularly those with OSA, are predisposed to postoperative pulmonary complications, including atelectasis. This can be mitigated with chest physiotherapy and incentive spirometry. CPAP and NPPV in the first 24 h postoperatively may effectively restore lung volumes to the preoperative values in obese patients [7].

Obese patients have a large potential space after wound closure which is often poorly vascularised and predisposed to necrosis [98]. Surgical-site infection (SSI) in obese patients is more prevalent than in patients of normal BMI [1, 10, 11]. A meta-analysis has revealed a BMI >35 as the most reliable predictor of SSI after spinal surgery [99]. Other independent risk factors highlighted in this study were diabetes and longer operative times (>3 h). SSI has been linked with long-term increased back pain and a lesser chance of achieving the minimum clinically important difference [100]. Specific care bundles in high-risk patients have been shown to reduce the rate of SSI following spine surgery [76]. Conventional strategies to reduce SSI include smoking cessation, tight glycaemic control, nasal/body decontamination, and nutritional optimisation. Application of local vancomycin powder is common practice among many spine surgeons due to a significant body of largely retrospective evidence [101, 102]. This practice has been challenged on the grounds of antimicrobial stewardship. Prior studies calculate a number needed to treat of 36 [103], and a more recent meta-analysis found that local vancomycin powder doubles the risk of Gram-negative or polymicrobial postoperative infection [104]. Prospective evidence for this treatment is conflicting [105, 106], and authors suggest that local vancomycin should be restricted only to patients who are most are risk [104].

There is a sevenfold greater risk of type 2 diabetes in people with obesity compared to normal BMI [107]. Wound infection rates following lumbar surgery have been reported to be approximately 10% in patients with diabetes [108]. Japanese researchers have found a negative correlation between recovery rate, as assessed via the Japanese Orthopaedic Association (JOA) score, and preoperative HbA1c in patients undergoing cervical expansive laminoplasty (OR 2.591; $p = 0.0193$) [109]. Elsewhere, retrospective database analysis was used to compare controlled versus uncontrolled DM complication rates following degenerative spinal surgery. Uncontrolled DM had increased odds of cardiac complications, deep vein thrombosis and postoperative shock, increased length of stay (average 5 days), and greater risk of inpatient mortality (OR = 6.39 CI 4.09–10.00 $P < 0.0001$) [110]. The above findings would suggest preoperative diabetes management warrants special consideration and tighter glycaemic control could yield more favourable surgical outcomes. Furthermore, HbA1c may be used as a prognostic marker for patient outcome in spinal surgery.

VTE is a relatively rare complication of elective spine surgery [111]; however, meta-analyses have found a higher rate of venous thromboembolism in obese patients recovering from spinal surgery than non-obese patients (OR 3.15; 95%CI, 1.92–5.17) [82]. When considering Virchow's triad, obesity has a role to play in each of hypercoagulability due to the pro-coagulant inflammatory process [28], and venous stasis due to immobility and endothelial damage indirectly caused by inflammatory mediators [28] and caused directly by surgery itself. Spine surgeons are tasked with balancing the risk of pulmonary embolism (PE) against the risk of permanent neurological damage from epidural haematoma. Chemoprophylaxis is for this reason contentious. A meta-analysis of 28 studies showed that the mean difference in the incidence of DVT and PE after spine surgery was not statistically significant when comparing mechanical prophylaxis (DVT 1%, PE 0.81%) with chemoprophylaxis (DVT 0.85%, PE 0.58%) [112]. The authors still acknowledge the role of chemoprophylaxis given the relatively high rate of fatal PE in their investigation (6% of PE's fatal).

6.7.2 Revision Surgeries

A meta-analysis of outcomes after spine surgery reports reoperation rates are higher in obese patients (OR 1.43; 95%CI 1.05–1.93) [82]. Subgroup analysis from the Spine Patient Outcome Research Trial (SPORT) illustrates that obese patients undergoing surgery for degenerative spondylolisthesis (DS) have twice the reoperation rate than that of non-obese patients at 4-year follow-up (20% vs. 11%, $P = 0.01$) [38]. SPORT was a randomised clinical trial which enrolled patients over 4 years from 13 multidisciplinary spine centres in 11 US states to compare the outcomes of surgical and non-operative treatment for DS, lumbar intervertebral disk herniation, and spinal stenosis (SS) [113]. Revision spinal surgeries are often technically difficult and exert a marked financial burden on the healthcare system. So too are they costly in psychological terms for patients and their families.

6.7.3 Functional Outcomes

Obesity's influence on functional and long-term clinical outcomes is controversial. The SPORT data found less improvement from baseline in the Short-Form 36 (SF-36) physical function score in obese patients after surgery for DS (22.6 vs. 27.9 $P = 0.022$) but no difference in clinical outcomes following surgery for lumbar spinal stenosis when comparing obese and non-obese patients [38]. Knutsson et al. noted that obese patients have worse Oswestry Disability Index (ODI), 33 vs. 25, and EuroQol five dimension Index (ED-5D), 0.56 vs. 0.64, than normal BMI patients and less mean improvement 2 years after surgery for lumbar spinal stenosis [114]. Wilson et al. demonstrated that obesity was associated with increased neck disability 1 year following surgery for degenerative cervical myelopathy [115].

However, conflicting evidence suggests no significant difference in pain and functional outcomes between obese and non-obese patients following lumbar spinal fusion [116]. Ghobrial et al. found no difference between obese and non-obese patient outcomes following non-instrumented lumbar surgery [117]. Furthermore, Myllykangas et al. found that there are no differences in quality of life as measured by ED-5D and ODI in obese versus non-obese postoperatively for lumbar spinal stenosis [11]. These findings are difficult to synthesise, and perhaps the reason for this controversy is the relatively limited body of research in the subject area [116]. Obese patients considering spine surgery should be advised of the conflicting evidence around long-term functional outcomes and expectations should be measured appropriately.

6.8 Conclusion

At present, obesity demands special consideration from spine services. One can expect these demands to trend upwards as the prevalence of obesity continues to rise. The evidence around functional outcomes following spine surgery in obese patients is conflicting, but is not convincing to suggest that patients should be excluded from surgical consideration on the basis of size alone. Careful preoperative planning is fundamental to surgical success in this objectively challenging patient cohort. Alignment of bariatric services alongside spinal services may be a solution to increasing the impact of the preoperative period in the obese patient group. Intraoperative advances in minimally invasive techniques including computer navigation and robotics are likely to help with the technical challenges of operating on the obese spine. These technologies are however in their infancy and will need to become more widely available before seeing their effect on spinal surgery in obese patients. The postoperative period in the obese cohort is challenging in terms of delayed mobilisation and subsequent complications. However, many of these complications can be lessened through the tailored approach to care both preoperatively and intraoperatively. The body of research around obesity and spinal surgery can be expected to grow substantially in the coming years, with more and more spinal services adapting their practices to facilitate the growing obese population.

Key Points

- Obesity is fundamentally linked to degenerative spinal pathology.
- Obese patients present specific challenges throughout all points of the perioperative period.
- Careful preoperative planning is fundamental to surgical success in this patient cohort.
- Preoperative bariatric surgery may be of particular benefit in obese patients requiring elective spinal procedures.
- Obese patients should not be excluded from surgical consideration on the basis of BMI alone.
- Advances in minimally invasive surgery, computer navigation, and robotics may support spinal surgery in obese patients, but these technologies are still in their infancy.

References

1. Jensen MD, Ryan DH, Apovian CM, et al. 2013 AHA/ACC/TOS guideline for the management of overweight and obesity in adults: a report of the American College of Cardiology/American Heart Association Task Force on Practice Guidelines and The Obesity Society. Circulation. 2014;129(25 Suppl 2):S102–38. https://doi.org/10.1161/01.cir.0000437739.71477.ee.
2. Walid MS, Robinson JS. Economic impact of comorbidities in spine surgery: clinical article. J Neurosurg Spine. 2011;14(3):318–21. https://doi.org/10.3171/2010.11.Spine10139.
3. Samartzis D, Karppinen J, Chan D, Luk KD, Cheung KM. The association of lumbar intervertebral disc degeneration on magnetic resonance imaging with body mass index in overweight and obese adults: a population-based study. Arthritis Rheum. 2012;64(5):1488–96. https://doi.org/10.1002/art.33462.
4. Su CA, Kusin DJ, Li SQ, Ahn UM, Ahn NU. The association between body mass index and the prevalence, severity, and frequency of low back pain: data from the osteoarthritis initiative. Spine (Phila Pa 1976). 2018;43(12):848–52.
5. Kauppila LI. Atherosclerosis and disc degeneration/low-back pain—a systematic review. Eur J Vasc Endovasc Surg. 2009;37(6):661–70. https://doi.org/10.1016/j.ejvs.2009.02.006.
6. Solovieva S, Lohiniva J, Leino-Arjas P, et al. COL9A3 gene polymorphism and obesity in intervertebral disc degeneration of the lumbar spine: evidence of gene-

environment interaction. Spine (Phila Pa 1976). 2002;27(23):2691–6. https://doi.org/10.1097/00007632-200212010-00008.
7. Pelosi P, Gregoretti C. Perioperative management of obese patients. Best Pract Res Clin Anaesthesiol. 2010;24(2):211–25. https://doi.org/10.1016/j.bpa.2010.02.001.
8. Brodsky JB. Recent advances in anesthesia of the obese patient. F1000Res. 2018;7:F1000 Faculty Rev-1195. https://doi.org/10.12688/f1000research.15093.1.
9. Khanna P, Sarkar S, Garg B. Anesthetic considerations in spine surgery: what orthopaedic surgeon should know! J Clin Orthop Trauma. 2020;11(5):742–8. https://doi.org/10.1016/j.jcot.2020.05.005.
10. Ortiz VE, Kwo J. Obesity: physiologic changes and implications for preoperative management. BMC Anesthesiol. 2015;15(1):97. https://doi.org/10.1186/s12871-015-0079-8.
11. Myllykangas H, Ristolainen L, Hurri H, et al. Obese people benefit from lumbar spinal stenosis surgery as much as people of normal weight. J Orthop Surg Res. 2021;16(1):550. https://doi.org/10.1186/s13018-021-02692-z.
12. Qin R, Liu B, Hao J, et al. Percutaneous endoscopic lumbar discectomy versus posterior open lumbar microdiscectomy for the treatment of symptomatic lumbar disc herniation: a systemic review and meta-analysis. World Neurosurg. 2018;120:352–62. https://doi.org/10.1016/j.wneu.2018.08.236.
13. Ruetten S, Komp M, Godolias G. A new full-endoscopic technique for the interlaminar operation of lumbar disc herniations using 6-mm endoscopes: prospective 2-year results of 331 patients. Minim Invasive Neurosurg. 2006;49(2):80–7. https://doi.org/10.1055/s-2006-932172.
14. Ahn Y, Lee S, Son S, Kim H. Learning curve for interlaminar endoscopic lumbar discectomy: a systematic review. World Neurosurg. 2021;150:93–100. https://doi.org/10.1016/j.wneu.2021.03.128.
15. Shafi KA, Pompeu YA, Vaishnav AS, et al. Does robot-assisted navigation influence pedicle screw selection and accuracy in minimally invasive spine surgery? Neurosurg Focus. 2022;52(1):E4. https://doi.org/10.3171/2021.10.Focus21526.
16. Zhang Q, Fan MX, Han XG, et al. Risk factors of unsatisfactory robot-assisted pedicle screw placement: a case-control study. Neurospine. 2021;18(4):839–44. https://doi.org/10.14245/ns.2142560.180.
17. Yang BP, Wahl MM, Idler CS. Percutaneous lumbar pedicle screw placement aided by computer-assisted fluoroscopy-based navigation: perioperative results of a prospective, comparative, multicenter study. Spine (Phila Pa 1976). 2012;37(24):2055–60. https://doi.org/10.1097/BRS.0b013e31825c05cd.
18. Fan Y, Du JP, Liu JJ, et al. Accuracy of pedicle screw placement comparing robot-assisted technology and the free-hand with fluoroscopy-guided method in spine surgery: an updated meta-analysis. Medicine (Baltimore). 2018;97(22):e10970. https://doi.org/10.1097/md.0000000000010970.
19. D'Souza M, Gendreau J, Feng A, Kim LH, Ho AL, Veeravagu A. Robotic-assisted spine surgery: history, efficacy, cost, and future trends. Robot Surg. 2019;6:9–23. https://doi.org/10.2147/rsrr.S190720.
20. Roser F, Tatagiba M, Maier G. Spinal robotics: current applications and future perspectives. Neurosurgery. 2013;72(Suppl 1):A12–8. https://doi.org/10.1227/NEU.0b013e318270d02c.
21. https://www-sciencedirect-com.ucd.idm.oclc.org/science/article/pii/S1878875018327499?via%3Dihub.
22. Zhang JN, Fan Y, Hao DJ. Risk factors for robot-assisted spinal pedicle screw malposition. Sci Rep. 2019;9(1):3025. https://doi.org/10.1038/s41598-019-40057-z.
23. Jacobsen S, Sonne-Holm S, Rovsing H, Monrad H, Gebuhr P. Degenerative lumbar spondylolisthesis: an epidemiological perspective: the Copenhagen Osteoarthritis Study. Spine (Phila Pa 1976). 2007;32(1):120–5.
24. Knutsson B, Sandén B, Sjödén G, Järvholm B, Michaëlsson K. Body mass index and risk for clinical lumbar spinal stenosis: a cohort study. Spine (Phila Pa 1976). 2015;40(18):1451–6.

25. Schroeder GD, Guyre CA, Vaccaro AR. The epidemiology and pathophysiology of lumbar disc herniations. Semin Spine Surg. 2016;28(1):2–7. https://doi.org/10.1053/j.semss.2015.08.003.
26. Wang T, He C. Pro-inflammatory cytokines: the link between obesity and osteoarthritis. Cytokine Growth Factor Rev. 2018;44:38–50. https://doi.org/10.1016/j.cytogfr.2018.10.002.
27. Carman WJ, Sowers M, Hawthorne VM, Weissfeld LA. Obesity as a risk factor for osteoarthritis of the hand and wrist: a prospective study. Am J Epidemiol. 1994;139(2):119–29. https://doi.org/10.1093/oxfordjournals.aje.a116974.
28. Balistreri CR, Caruso C, Candore G. The role of adipose tissue and adipokines in obesity-related inflammatory diseases. Mediat Inflamm. 2010;2010:802078. https://doi.org/10.1155/2010/802078.
29. Zhao C-Q, Liu D, Li H, Jiang L-S, Dai L-Y. Expression of leptin and its functional receptor on disc cells: contribution to cell proliferation. Spine (Phila Pa 1976). 2008;33(23):E858–64.
30. Pottie P, Presle N, Dumond H, et al. Is leptin the link between obesity and osteoarthritis? Arthritis Res Ther. 2004;6(3):8. https://doi.org/10.1186/ar1342.
31. Dumond H, Presle N, Terlain B, et al. Evidence for a key role of leptin in osteoarthritis. Arthritis Rheum. 2003;48(11):3118–29. https://doi.org/10.1002/art.11303.
32. Eskola PJ, Lemmelä S, Kjaer P, et al. Genetic association studies in lumbar disc degeneration: a systematic review. PLoS One. 2012;7(11):e49995. https://doi.org/10.1371/journal.pone.0049995.
33. Schelbert KB. Comorbidities of obesity. Prim Care. 2009;36(2):271–85. https://doi.org/10.1016/j.pop.2009.01.009.
34. North American Spine Society. Diagnosis & Treatment of Low Back Pain. 2020. Evidence-based clinical guidelines for multidisciplinary spine care. https://www.spine.org/Research-Clinical-Care/Quality-Improvement/Clinical-Guidelines.
35. Hahne AJ, Ford JJ, McMeeken JM. Conservative management of lumbar disc herniation with associated radiculopathy: a systematic review. Spine (Phila Pa 1976). 2010;35(11):E488–504.
36. Wasser JG, Vasilopoulos T, Zdziarski LA, Vincent HK. Exercise benefits for chronic low back pain in overweight and obese individuals. PM&R. 2017;9(2):181–92. https://doi.org/10.1016/j.pmrj.2016.06.019.
37. McGuire KJ, Khaleel MA, Rihn JA, Lurie JD, Zhao W, Weinstein JN. The effect of high obesity on outcomes of treatment for lumbar spinal conditions: subgroup analysis of the spine patient outcomes research trial. Spine (Phila Pa 1976). 2014;39(23):1975–80. https://doi.org/10.1097/BRS.0000000000000577.
38. Rihn JA, Radcliff K, Hilibrand AS, et al. Does obesity affect outcomes of treatment for lumbar stenosis and degenerative spondylolisthesis? Analysis of the Spine Patient Outcomes Research Trial (SPORT). Spine (Phila Pa 1976). 2012;37(23):1933–46. https://doi.org/10.1097/BRS.0b013e31825e21b2.
39. North American Spine Society. Clinical Guidelines for Diagnosis and Treatment of Lumbar Disc Herniation with Radiculopathy. 2012. Evidence-based clinical guidelines for multidisciplinary spine care. https://www.spine.org/Research-Clinical-Care/Quality-Improvement/Clinical-Guidelines.
40. McCormick Z, Plastaras C. Lumbosacral transforaminal epidural steroid injections are equally effective for treatment of lumbosacral radicular pain in the obese compared to non-obese population: a pilot study. J Back Musculoskelet Rehabil. 2013;26(2):183–8. https://doi.org/10.3233/bmr-130366.
41. Chew I, De Souza R, Reisch J, Le J. Efficacy of lumbar epidural steroid injections for lumbosacral radiculopathy in individuals with obesity: a retrospective comparative study. Intervent Pain Med. 2022;1(3):100109. https://doi.org/10.1016/j.inpm.2022.100109.
42. Chou R, Qaseem A, Owens DK, Shekelle P. Diagnostic imaging for low back pain: advice for high-value health care from the American College of Physicians. Ann Intern Med. 2011;154(3):181–9. https://doi.org/10.7326/0003-4819-154-3-201102010-00008.

43. McCormick ZL, Choxi SC, Lee DT, et al. The impact of body mass index on fluoroscopy time during lumbar epidural steroid injection; a multicenter cohort study. Pain Med. 2017;18(1):25–35. https://doi.org/10.1093/pm/pnw050.
44. Mann SD, Joshi A, Shonyo M, et al. Improved dose estimates for fluoroscopically guided lumbar epidural injections. Pain Med. 2018;20(5):971–8. https://doi.org/10.1093/pm/pny172.
45. Al-Khawaja D, Seex K, Eslick GD. Spinal epidural lipomatosis—a brief review. J Clin Neurosci. 2008;15(12):1323–6. https://doi.org/10.1016/j.jocn.2008.03.001.
46. Theyskens NC, Paulino Pereira NR, Janssen SJ, Bono CM, Schwab JH, Cha TD. The prevalence of spinal epidural lipomatosis on magnetic resonance imaging. Spine J. 2017;17(7):969–76. https://doi.org/10.1016/j.spinee.2017.02.010.
47. Jaimes R, Rocco AG. Multiple epidural steroid injections and body mass index linked with occurrence of epidural lipomatosis: a case series. BMC Anesthesiol. 2014;14(1):70. https://doi.org/10.1186/1471-2253-14-70.
48. Fassett DR, Schmidt MH. Spinal epidural lipomatosis: a review of its causes and recommendations for treatment. J Neurosurg. 2004;16(4):1–3. https://doi.org/10.3171/foc.2004.16.4.12.
49. Tok CH, Kaur S, Gangi A. Symptomatic spinal epidural lipomatosis after a single local epidural steroid injection. Cardiovasc Intervent Radiol. 2011;34(2):250–5. https://doi.org/10.1007/s00270-010-9982-z.
50. McCullen GM, Spurling GR, Webster JS. Epidural lipomatosis complicating lumbar steroid injections. J Spinal Disord. 1999;12(6):526–9.
51. Sandberg DI, Lavyne MH. Symptomatic spinal epidural lipomatosis after local epidural corticosteroid injections: case report. Neurosurgery. 1999;45(1):162–5. https://doi.org/10.1097/00006123-199907000-00037.
52. Gerber P, Anderin C, Thorell A. Weight loss prior to bariatric surgery: an updated review of the literature. Scand J Surg. 2015;104(1):33–9. https://doi.org/10.1177/1457496914553149.
53. Nielsen PR, Jørgensen LD, Dahl B, Pedersen T, Tønnesen H. Prehabilitation and early rehabilitation after spinal surgery: randomized clinical trial. Clin Rehabil. 2010;24(2):137–48. https://doi.org/10.1177/0269215509347432.
54. Roffey DM, Ashdown LC, Dornan HD, et al. Pilot evaluation of a multidisciplinary, medically supervised, nonsurgical weight loss program on the severity of low back pain in obese adults. Spine J. 2011;11(3):197–204. https://doi.org/10.1016/j.spinee.2011.01.031.
55. Garcia Ulen C, Huizinga MM, Beech B, Elasy TA. Weight regain prevention. Clin Diabetes. 2008;26(3):100–13. https://doi.org/10.2337/diaclin.26.3.100.
56. Gometz A, Maislen D, Youtz C, et al. The effectiveness of prehabilitation (prehab) in both functional and economic outcomes following spinal surgery: a systematic review. Cureus. 2018;10(5):e2675. https://doi.org/10.7759/cureus.2675.
57. Debono B, Wainwright TW, Wang MY, et al. Consensus statement for perioperative care in lumbar spinal fusion: Enhanced Recovery After Surgery (ERAS®) Society recommendations. Spine J. 2021;21(5):729–52. https://doi.org/10.1016/j.spinee.2021.01.001.
58. Maciejewski ML, Arterburn DE, Van Scoyoc L, et al. Bariatric surgery and long-term durability of weight loss. JAMA Surg. 2016;151(11):1046–55. https://doi.org/10.1001/jamasurg.2016.2317.
59. Khoueir P, Black MH, Crookes PF, Kaufman HS, Katkhouda N, Wang MY. Prospective assessment of axial back pain symptoms before and after bariatric weight reduction surgery. Spine J. 2009;9(6):454–63. https://doi.org/10.1016/j.spinee.2009.02.003.
60. Robinson MK. Surgical treatment of obesity—weighing the facts. N Engl J Med. 2009;361(5):520–1. https://doi.org/10.1056/NEJMe0904837.
61. Koremans FW, Chen X, Das A, Diwan AD. Changes in back pain scores after bariatric surgery in obese patients: a systematic review and meta-analysis. J Clin Med. 2021;10(7):1443. https://doi.org/10.3390/jcm10071443.
62. Passias PG, Alas H, Kummer N, et al. Bariatric surgery diminishes spinal diagnoses in a morbidly obese population: a 2-year survivorship analysis of cervical and lumbar pathologies. J Clin Neurosci. 2021;90:135–9. https://doi.org/10.1016/j.jocn.2021.05.012.

63. Passias PG, Horn SR, Vasquez-Montes D, et al. Prior bariatric surgery lowers complication rates following spine surgery in obese patients. Acta Neurochir. 2018;160(12):2459–65. https://doi.org/10.1007/s00701-018-3722-6.
64. Alhammoud A, Dalal S, Sheha ED, et al. The impact of prior bariatric surgery on outcomes after spine surgery: a systematic review and meta-analysis. Global Spine J. 2022;12(8):1872–80. https://doi.org/10.1177/21925682211072492.
65. Malik AT, Noria S, Xu W, Retchin S, Yu ES, Khan SN. Bariatric surgery before elective anterior cervical discectomy and fusion (ACDF) in obese patients is associated with reduced risk of 90-day postoperative complications and readmissions. Clin Spine Surg. 2021;34(5):171–5. https://doi.org/10.1097/bsd.0000000000001120.
66. McLawhorn AS, Levack AE, Lee YY, Ge Y, Do H, Dodwell ER. Bariatric surgery improves outcomes after lower extremity arthroplasty in the morbidly obese: a propensity score-matched analysis of a New York statewide database. J Arthroplast. 2018;33(7):2062–9.e4. https://doi.org/10.1016/j.arth.2017.11.056.
67. Stein EM, Carrelli A, Young P, et al. Bariatric surgery results in cortical bone loss. J Clin Endocrinol Metab. 2013;98(2):541–9. https://doi.org/10.1210/jc.2012-2394.
68. Wei JH, Lee WJ, Chong K, et al. High incidence of secondary hyperparathyroidism in bariatric patients: comparing different procedures. Obes Surg. 2018;28(3):798–804. https://doi.org/10.1007/s11695-017-2932-y.
69. Zhang Q, Chen Y, Li J, et al. A meta-analysis of the effects of bariatric surgery on fracture risk. Obes Rev. 2018;19(5):728–36. https://doi.org/10.1111/obr.12665.
70. Makras P, Anastasilakis AD. Bone disease in primary hyperparathyroidism. Metabolism. 2018;80:57–65. https://doi.org/10.1016/j.metabol.2017.10.003.
71. Yu EW. Bone metabolism after bariatric surgery. J Bone Miner Res. 2014;29(7):1507–18. https://doi.org/10.1002/jbmr.2226.
72. Uppot RN. Technical challenges of imaging & image-guided interventions in obese patients. Br J Radiol. 2018;91(1089):20170931. https://doi.org/10.1259/bjr.20170931.
73. Modica MJ, Kanal KM, Gunn ML. The obese emergency patient: imaging challenges and solutions. Radiographics. 2011;31(3):811–23. https://doi.org/10.1148/rg.313105138.
74. Sessler DI. Temperature monitoring and perioperative thermoregulation. Anesthesiology. 2008;109(2):318–38. https://doi.org/10.1097/ALN.0b013e31817f6d76.
75. Yi J, Xiang Z, Deng X, et al. Incidence of inadvertent intraoperative hypothermia and its risk factors in patients undergoing general anesthesia in Beijing: a prospective regional survey. PLoS One. 2015;10(9):e0136136. https://doi.org/10.1371/journal.pone.0136136.
76. Aleem IS, Tan LA, Nassr A, Riew KD. Surgical site infection prevention following spine surgery. Global Spine J. 2020;10(1 Suppl):92s–8s. https://doi.org/10.1177/2192568219844228.
77. Okoué R, Calabrese D, Nzé P, Msika S, Keita H. Efficacy of forced-air warming to prevent perioperative hypothermia in morbidly-obese versus non-obese patients. Obes Surg. 2018;28(7):1955–9. https://doi.org/10.1007/s11695-017-3108-5.
78. Riley C, Andrzejowski J. Inadvertent perioperative hypothermia. BJA Educ. 2018;18(8):227–33. https://doi.org/10.1016/j.bjae.2018.05.003.
79. Lenhardt R, Marker E, Goll V, et al. Mild intraoperative hypothermia prolongs postanesthetic recovery. Anesthesiology. 1997;87(6):1318–23. https://doi.org/10.1097/00000542-199712000-00009.
80. Buraimoh MA, Nash A, Howard B, et al. Effect of forced-air warming blanket position in elective lumbar spine surgery: intraoperative body temperature and postoperative complications. Surg Neurol Int. 2019;10:229. https://doi.org/10.25259/sni_102_2019.
81. Moola S, Lockwood C. Effectiveness of strategies for the management and/or prevention of hypothermia within the adult perioperative environment. Int J Evid Based Healthc. 2011;9(4):337–45. https://doi.org/10.1111/j.1744-1609.2011.00227.x.
82. Jiang J, Teng Y, Fan Z, Khan S, Xia Y. Does obesity affect the surgical outcome and complication rates of spinal surgery? A meta-analysis. Clin Orthop Relat Res. 2014;472(3):968–75. https://doi.org/10.1007/s11999-013-3346-3.

83. Han IH, Son DW, Nam KH, Choi BK, Song GS. The effect of body mass index on intra-abdominal pressure and blood loss in lumbar spine surgery. J Korean Neurosurg Soc. 2012;51(2):81–5. https://doi.org/10.3340/jkns.2012.51.2.81.
84. DePasse JM, Palumbo MA, Haque M, Eberson CP, Daniels AH. Complications associated with prone positioning in elective spinal surgery. World J Orthop. 2015;6(3):351–9. https://doi.org/10.5312/wjo.v6.i3.351.
85. Chang SH, Miller NR. The incidence of vision loss due to perioperative ischemic optic neuropathy associated with spine surgery: the Johns Hopkins Hospital experience. Spine (Phila Pa 1976). 2005;30(11):1299–302. https://doi.org/10.1097/01.brs.0000163884.11476.25.
86. Kundra S, Bansal H, Gupta V, et al. A comparative evaluation of the effect of prone positioning methods on blood loss and intra-abdominal pressure in obese patients undergoing spinal surgery. J Neuroanaesth Crit Care. 2021;8(02):92–8.
87. Rosenfeld HE, Limb R, Chan P, Fitzgerald M, Pierre W, Rosenfeld JV. Challenges in the surgical management of spine trauma in the morbidly obese patient: a case series. J Neurosurg Spine. 2013;19(1):101–9. https://doi.org/10.3171/2013.4.spine12876.
88. Bochicchio GV, Joshi M, Bochicchio K, Nehman S, Kathleen Tracy J, Scalea TM. Impact of obesity in the critically ill trauma patient: a prospective study. J Am Coll Surg. 2006;203(4):533–8. https://doi.org/10.1016/j.jamcollsurg.2006.07.001.
89. Momin AA, Steinmetz MP. Evolution of minimally invasive lumbar spine surgery. World Neurosurg. 2020;140:622–6. https://doi.org/10.1016/j.wneu.2020.05.071.
90. Hammad A, Wirries A, Ardeshiri A, Nikiforov O, Geiger F. Open versus minimally invasive TLIF: literature review and meta-analysis. J Orthop Surg Res. 2019;14(1):229. https://doi.org/10.1186/s13018-019-1266-y.
91. Tan JH, Liu G, Ng R, Kumar N, Wong HK, Liu G. Is MIS-TLIF superior to open TLIF in obese patients?: a systematic review and meta-analysis. Eur Spine J. 2018;27(8):1877–86. https://doi.org/10.1007/s00586-018-5630-0.
92. Mueller K, Zhao D, Johnson O, Sandhu FA, Voyadzis JM. The difference in surgical site infection rates between open and minimally invasive spine surgery for degenerative lumbar pathology: a retrospective single center experience of 1442 cases. Oper Neurosurg (Hagerstown). 2019;16(6):750–5. https://doi.org/10.1093/ons/opy221.
93. Price JP, Dawson JM, Schwender JD, Schellhas KP. Clinical and radiologic comparison of minimally invasive surgery with traditional open transforaminal lumbar interbody fusion: a review of 452 patients from a single center. Clin Spine Surg. 2018;31(2):E121–6. https://doi.org/10.1097/bsd.0000000000000581.
94. Mao JZ, Agyei JO, Khan A, et al. Technologic evolution of navigation and robotics in spine surgery: a historical perspective. World Neurosurg. 2021;145:159–67. https://doi.org/10.1016/j.wneu.2020.08.224.
95. Wang D, Teddy PJ, Henderson NJ, Shine BS, Gardner BP. Mobilization of patients after spinal surgery for acute spinal cord injury. Spine (Phila Pa 1976). 2001;26(20):2278–82. https://doi.org/10.1097/00007632-200110150-00022.
96. Burks CA, Werner BC, Yang S, Shimer AL. Obesity is associated with an increased rate of incidental durotomy in lumbar spine surgery. Spine (Phila Pa 1976). 2015;40(7):500–4. https://doi.org/10.1097/brs.0000000000000784.
97. Verma K, Freelin AH, Atkinson KA, Graham RS, Broaddus WC. Early mobilization versus bed rest for incidental durotomy: an institutional cohort study. J Neurosurg Spine. 2022;37(3):460–5. https://doi.org/10.3171/2022.1.Spine211208.
98. Massie JB, Heller JG, Abitbol JJ, McPherson D, Garfin SR. Postoperative posterior spinal wound infections. Clin Orthop Relat Res. 1992;284:99–108.
99. Fei Q, Li J, Lin J, et al. Risk factors for surgical site infection after spinal surgery: a meta-analysis. World Neurosurg. 2016;95:507–15. https://doi.org/10.1016/j.wneu.2015.05.059.
100. Petilon JM, Glassman SD, Dimar JR, Carreon LY. Clinical outcomes after lumbar fusion complicated by deep wound infection: a case-control study. Spine (Phila Pa 1976). 2012;37(16):1370–4. https://doi.org/10.1097/BRS.0b013e31824a4d93.

101. Hey HWD, Thiam DW, Koh ZSD, et al. Is intraoperative local vancomycin powder the answer to surgical site infections in spine surgery? Spine (Phila Pa 1976). 2017;42(4):267–74. https://doi.org/10.1097/brs.0000000000001710.
102. Ghobrial GM, Cadotte DW, Williams K, Fehlings MG, Harrop JS. Complications from the use of intrawound vancomycin in lumbar spinal surgery: a systematic review. Neurosurgical Focus FOC. 2015;39(4):E11. https://doi.org/10.3171/2015.7.Focus15258.
103. Khan NR, Thompson CJ, DeCuypere M, et al. A meta-analysis of spinal surgical site infection and vancomycin powder: a review. J Neurosurg Spine. 2014;21(6):974–83. https://doi.org/10.3171/2014.8.Spine1445.
104. Gande A, Rosinski A, Cunningham T, Bhatia N, Lee YP. Selection pressures of vancomycin powder use in spine surgery: a meta-analysis. Spine J. 2019;19(6):1076–84. https://doi.org/10.1016/j.spinee.2019.01.002.
105. Salimi S, Khayat Kashani HR, Azhari S, et al. Local vancomycin therapy to reduce surgical site infection in adult spine surgery: a randomized prospective study. Eur Spine J. 2022;31(2):454–60. https://doi.org/10.1007/s00586-021-07050-5.
106. Tubaki VR, Rajasekaran S, Shetty AP. Effects of using intravenous antibiotic only versus local intrawound vancomycin antibiotic powder application in addition to intravenous antibiotics on postoperative infection in spine surgery in 907 patients. Spine (Phila Pa 1976). 2013;38(25):2149–55. https://doi.org/10.1097/brs.0000000000000015.
107. Abdullah A, Peeters A, de Courten M, Stoelwinder J. The magnitude of association between overweight and obesity and the risk of diabetes: a meta-analysis of prospective cohort studies. Diabetes Res Clin Pract. 2010;89(3):309–19. https://doi.org/10.1016/j.diabres.2010.04.012.
108. Simpson JM, Silveri CP, Balderston RA, Simeone FA, An HS. The results of operations on the lumbar spine in patients who have diabetes mellitus. J Bone Joint Surg Am. 1993;75(12):1823–9. https://doi.org/10.2106/00004623-199312000-00013.
109. Machino M, Yukawa Y, Ito K, et al. Risk factors for poor outcome of cervical laminoplasty for cervical spondylotic myelopathy in patients with diabetes. JBJS. 2014;96(24):2049–55. https://doi.org/10.2106/jbjs.N.00064.
110. Guzman JZ, Skovrlj B, Shin J, et al. The impact of diabetes mellitus on patients undergoing degenerative cervical spine surgery. Spine (Phila Pa 1976). 2014;39(20):1656–65. https://doi.org/10.1097/brs.0000000000000498.
111. Bono CM, Watters WC 3rd, Heggeness MH, et al. An evidence-based clinical guideline for the use of antithrombotic therapies in spine surgery. Spine J. 2009;9(12):1046–51. https://doi.org/10.1016/j.spinee.2009.09.005.
112. Mosenthal WP, Landy DC, Boyajian HH, et al. Thromboprophylaxis in spinal surgery. Spine (Phila Pa 1976). 2018;43(8):E474–81. https://doi.org/10.1097/brs.0000000000002379.
113. Weinstein JN, Tosteson TD, Lurie JD, et al. Surgical versus nonoperative treatment for lumbar spinal stenosis four-year results of the spine patient outcomes research trial. Spine (Phila Pa 1976). 2010;35(14):1329–38. https://doi.org/10.1097/BRS.0b013e3181e0f04d.
114. Knutsson B, Michaëlsson K, Sandén B. Obesity is associated with inferior results after surgery for lumbar spinal stenosis: a study of 2633 patients from the Swedish spine register. Spine (Phila Pa 1976). 2013;38(5):435–41. https://doi.org/10.1097/BRS.0b013e318270b243.
115. Wilson JR, Tetreault LA, Schroeder G, et al. Impact of elevated body mass index and obesity on long-term surgical outcomes for patients with degenerative cervical myelopathy: analysis of a combined prospective dataset. Spine (Phila Pa 1976). 2017;42(3):195–201. https://doi.org/10.1097/brs.0000000000001859.
116. Lingutla KK, Pollock R, Benomran E, et al. Outcome of lumbar spinal fusion surgery in obese patients: a systematic review and meta-analysis. Bone Joint J. 2015;97-b(10):1395–404. https://doi.org/10.1302/0301-620x.97b10.35724.
117. Ghobrial J, Gadjradj P, Harhangi B, Dammers R, Vleggeert-Lankamp C. Outcome of non-instrumented lumbar spinal surgery in obese patients: a systematic review. Br J Neurosurg. 2021;36(4):447–56. https://doi.org/10.1080/02688697.2021.1885615.

7 Obesity and Osteoarthritis of the Hip

Peggy Miller, Alexander Vincent, and Colin Murphy

7.1 Introduction and Epidemiology

The relationship between obesity and osteoarthritis of the hip joint has been described extensively in the literature. In this chapter, we will discuss the role of obesity and osteoarthritic degeneration of the hip joint, considerations for total hip arthroplasty (THA) in obese patients, and postoperative complications and outcomes faced by these patients.

Obesity is defined by the World Health Organization as abnormal or excessive fat accumulation that may impair health. Obesity is often classified using body mass index (BMI) which is calculated by a person's weight in kilograms divided by the square of their height in metres (kg/m^2). BMI < 18 is considered underweight, 18–25.9 is considered normal or acceptable, 26–30 is overweight, obese class 1 is a BMI greater than 30, obese class 2 is greater than 35, and obese class 3 is greater than 40. Super-obese is considered a BMI greater than 50 [1].

Obesity is on the rise across the world. It is predicted that soon there will be more adults in the United States with an elevated BMI compared to those with a normal BMI of <26 [2]. A population prediction model of health suggests that by 2030 there will be an increase in the prevalence of obesity in the United States from 32% in 2008 to 50–51%, and from 26% to 35–43% in the United Kingdom [3]. This

P. Miller (✉)
University Hospital Waterford, Waterford, Ireland

Royal College of Surgeons Ireland, Dublin 2, Ireland

A. Vincent
Royal College of Surgeons Ireland, Dublin 2, Ireland
e-mail: Alexandervincent@rcsi.ie

C. Murphy
Galway University Hospital, Galway, Ireland
e-mail: Cmurphy@rcsi.ie

J. M. O´Byrne et al. (eds.), *Musculoskeletal Disease and Obesity*,
https://doi.org/10.1007/978-3-031-63310-2_7

research suggests that by 2030 there will be 65 million more obese adults in the United States than in 2010 and 11 million more in the United Kingdom. It is predicted that the increase in spending will be an additional $48–66 billion/year in the United States and £1.9–2 billion annually in the United Kingdom. The cost burden associated with this increase in obesity is largely attributed to the associated conditions or comorbidities associated with obesity, including type 2 diabetes mellitus, stroke, and cardiac health issues.

7.2 Osteoarthritis

Osteoarthritis (OA) is also linked to obesity. Osteoarthritis is defined as a degenerative joint disease involving loss of articular cartilage. It is the most common cause of chronic joint pain worldwide and is the leading cause of workplace absenteeism in working-age adults. The pathogenesis of osteoarthritis has no definitive cause; however, trauma, obesity, and occupation are established risk factors [4].

In weight-bearing joints, OA may be linked to both an inflammatory reaction to obesity or metabolic syndrome, and the increased mechanical loading on the joint. This is discussed in more detail in other areas of this book.

When considering mechanical loading and inflammatory reaction in the joint, it is unclear which predominates as the primary cause of hip osteoarthritis. Most likely it is both that will predispose an obese individual to osteoarthritis. This occurs as the alteration in mechanical load and abnormal gait cause increased impact to the joint loading, causing damage to the articular cartilage, including splitting of the extracellular matrix, increased cellular activity, reduced tissue hydration, and abnormalities in remodelling of the subchondral bone [5]. Sturmer et al. describe a link between bilateral knee osteoarthritis in the obese patient and generalised osteoarthritis including the hands, but not in the hip [6]. This suggests that the hip joint is more affected by increased mechanical load compared with the knee joint and less by the systemic reaction.

An increase in BMI, even within the range considered to be a normal, shows a linear relationship between osteoarthritis and increased weight as described by Järvholm et al. in a study on a population of young, male construction workers [7]. They found that workers with BMI = 20–24 were twice as likely to develop osteoarthritis compared with those with BMI = 17–19, despite both values being considered normal. This demonstrates that even modest increases in weight may have a negative impact on joint health.

By 2029 the number of patients in the obesity category undergoing total hip arthroplasty will increase from 36% in the years 1999–2019 to greater than 55% in 2029 [8]. Further research also suggests that patients under 25 years old who are obese may be predisposed to an increased risk for total hip arthroplasty later in life with an increased relative risk of 2.1 in men and an increased risk of 1.7 in women compared with their non-obese counterparts [9]. Many patients who will be undergoing THA for osteoarthritis of the hip later in life will be classified as obese. We will outline the special considerations for the treatment of these patients in this chapter.

7.3 Surgical Considerations

A trial of non-operative measures is completed prior to most surgical interventions. In hip osteoarthritis, this includes lifestyle alterations such as weight loss and non-weight-bearing exercise. Trials of simple analgesia and physiotherapy may also be considered, along with intra-articular corticosteroid injections. A patient will often follow this trajectory over several months to years and often with varying results. The definitive management of severe osteoarthritis of the hip impacting upon activities of daily living is a THA.

Appropriate patient selection is recognised as necessary in any type of surgery. Many considerations should be made in the preoperative management of a patient undergoing THA. Despite the obesity paradox (lower postoperative mortality rates in overweight and moderately obese patients undergoing surgery compared with patients of normal BMI or those who are underweight [10–12]), obesity is still considered a risk factor for a multitude of surgical complications including cardiorespiratory events, venous thromboembolic events, wound infections, increased length of stay, increased pain postoperatively, and increase risk of a prosthetic joint infection or prosthetic loosening in the context of a THA [13–15].

In this context obesity cutoff limits for surgical selection may be employed. Some studies have suggested that cutoff markers over a BMI of 40 or 50 may reduce surgical postop complications. These arbitrary cutoffs may be a healthcare systems' best chance to provide a utilitarian approach to rationing limited resources, given the enormous cost of treating these specific complications, but these policies may be considered biased and unfair as there is little difference in functional outcome or patient-reported outcome shown between patients who are obese and those who are not. Others have argued that these policies may act as a racist and sexist discrimination tool when selecting a surgical candidate as they have already been shown to negatively impact Black, Hispanic, and female patients in US studies [16, 17]. It has also been reported that obese patients undergo THA up to 10 years younger compared with their non-obese counterparts, thus highlighting the limitations imposed by cutoff criteria for surgery including age [18].

7.4 Preoperative Optimisation

Optimisation of these patients is advantageous before surgery. Studies have reviewed the role of pre-habilitation in elective surgery, but few specifically in obese patients. Education, exercise regimens, weight loss, and nutritional supplementation remain a 'mainstay' of the pre-habilitation course. The benefits of pre-habilitation for the patient and the health service include a reduced length of hospital stay and increased functional outcomes postop. This is relevant in the obese patient where the length of stay is increased post-THA [19]. The role of pre-habilitation before THA needs to be researched further to understand its role in the management of obese patients [20].

The role of the surgical treatment of obesity in the form of bariatric surgery may be an adjunct to preoperative optimisation. Weight loss is commonly recommended prior to an elective joint arthroplasty, but the role of bariatric surgery before total joint arthroplasty is yet to be fully evaluated. The relationship between the type of and length of time before surgery of bariatric surgery and postoperative complications following THA remains complex. Murr et al. report reductions in major and minor postoperative complications in this cohort, reduced operating room time, reduced length of hospital stay, decreased risk of re-operation, and reduced re-admission following total joint arthroplasty [21, 22]. When a patient requires bariatric surgery and THA, it is recommended that the patient undergo the bariatric intervention followed by the THA, with an optimal interval of at least 6 months [23]. Given the chronic metabolic state associated with obesity, the role of bariatric surgery in obesity is complex, and the role of this is unclear in the context of a THA. Having a patient undergo two major surgical interventions is a huge assault to a patient's immune and inflammatory system. Some studies have suggested higher rates of complications in obese patients undergoing THA following bariatric surgery. This raises questions about our understanding of the post-metabolic state and its related timing of arthroplasty [24–26].

7.5 Risks of Surgery

Performing total hip arthroplasty on obese patients poses an increased risk for both the patient and the surgical team. From a patient's perspective, heavier patients have an increased risk of airway complications, pressure areas, and neurovascular injuries. Similarly increased length of operating time and increased level of blood loss have been reported for obese patients. Obese patients with a BMI >30 lose an increased 380 mL of blood compared with a patient with BMI <26 [27], which has implications both for patient consent and perioperative transfusion risk.

7.6 Technical Considerations

Another consideration for surgeons when operating on obese patients is the surgical approach or technique. The surgical approach is most often based on surgeon experience and preference. The surgical approach for any patient is challenging due to the trade-off between the size of incision and exposure (larger incisions increase the risk of blood loss and increased risk of infection) as opposed to the risks due to insufficient visualisation of the surgical field (increased risk of fracture, neurovascular injury, malalignment, and malpositioning). Despite these concerns, it has been found that minimally invasive approaches benefit obese patients as much as patients of normal BMI in terms of time points of mobilisation, length of hospital stay, and functional outcome measurements [28]. With regard to component positioning, the risks of underanteversion or over-abduction of the acetabular component are reported to be much higher in morbidly obese patients [29] predisposing to elevated postoperative prosthesis-related complications.

Along with the perceived risk to the patient intraoperatively, there is also the risk to the staff and the surgical team. While orthopaedic surgery is considered a speciality with a high risk of occupational hazard [30], these risks could rise with increasing levels of obesity. Almost two-thirds of arthroplasty surgeons report a work-related injury including lumbar spine pain and lateral epicondylitis of the elbow most commonly, with 31% requiring surgical treatment of their injury [31, 32].

In an extensive survey of surgical ergonomics and musculoskeletal pain in arthroplasty surgeons, up to 96.5% experienced occupation-related musculoskeletal pain; this was statistically significant for height, weight, and BMI of the surgeon, but not for gender, running multiple operating rooms simultaneously, or annual caseload [33]. A positive correlation between burnout among surgeons and higher rates of musculoskeletal pain has been documented. While specific research evaluating the role of obesity in the surgical patient and occupational hazards to arthroplasty surgeons is lacking, it may be safe to suggest a negative relationship given prolonged operating time, poor posture of the surgeon, and the surgical team due to prolonged length of retraction time of heavier limbs. It is currently estimated that approximately 340 kcal/h are expended by the operating surgeon during a THA. This is higher than in a TKA. Longer surgeries require increased energy expenditure and thus may increase the risk of fatigue, dehydration, musculoskeletal injuries, and burnout among operating surgeons [34].

Consideration for all operating room staff in moving and assisting the obese patient must be considered and may require increased staffing levels and optimising manual handling to reduce the risk of injuries to staff and patients.

7.7 Surgical Outcomes

At the beginning of the last decade, much of the literature published surrounding postoperative complications following THA in obese patients described an increase in essentially all risks from the surgery. These include but are not limited to dislocation, infection, instability, deep vein thrombosis, pulmonary embolus, and sciatic nerve injury. Studies suggest an increased rate of complications up to fourfold in an obese patient compared with a patient who is not obese [35]. Multiple theories have been put forward as to why there may be an increased risk of complication, but as obesity is considered a chronic pro-inflammatory state, it may be an increase in this pro-inflammatory reaction in the perioperative period that increases these risks. A review of inflammatory marker levels postoperatively such as interleukin 1 and interleukin-6 along with TNF-alpha did not suggest an increase in this cytokine activity [36].

When considering infection in total joint arthroplasty, we consider superficial infection and also deep infections (PJI) causing septic loosening of a prosthesis. Studies have highlighted a link between superficial infections or wound-site infections and obesity [37]. It remains unclear, however, whether this link extends to septic loosening of a prosthesis, with certain studies reporting an increased risk in obese patients but others highlighting similar risk between obese and non-obese patients [38, 39]. The dosing of antibiotics in these patients still requires guidance, but we know that obesity causes increased volume distribution of antibiotics and alterations in hepatic and renal antibiotic metabolism [40]. Further research is necessary to ensure surgeons have appropriate guidance for antibiotic prophylaxis in these patients.

Dislocation is at increased risk in obese patients undergoing total hip arthroplasty; however, the extent of this remains unclear. Dislocation following THA is multifactorial, with surgeon-, patient-, and component-specific factors all relevant. Dislocation is thought to be at increased risk with cup anteversion and also inappropriate positioning postoperatively. Patients who are obese are more likely to be exposed to both of these risks which may account for some of the reported increased rate of dislocation.

Surgical approach is another consideration when undertaking THA. Posterior, lateral, and direct anterior are the most common approaches used for THA. Regarding the surgical approach in obese patients; it has been suggested in numerous studies that the direct anterior approach has a higher rate of infection in obese patients compared with the lateral and posterior [41–43]. Obese patients undergoing direct anterior approach were 3.6 times more likely to have a wound infection when compared with non-obese patients [44]. The suggested reasoning for this is the proximity to the inguinal folds in the DA approach. However, it may be argued that femoral head size is a more important factor in dislocation rates in obese patients than the surgical approach [45]. Consideration for component selection is often challenging; the decision regarding femoral head size (in order to try and reduce dislocation risk by increasing jump distance) at the cost of increased volumetric polyethylene wear in younger, heavier patients. Intraoperative sizing is recommended, along with the use of dual mobility and constrained liners [46]. Dual mobility-type bearing surfaces have been found to mitigate the risk of dislocation even in obese patients [47]. There is evidence of efficacy and implant survival at the 10-year postop point [48]. Further research into this area will be useful to understand why this may be higher in obese patients and in the context of other factors such as gender [49].

Osteolysis is defined as the process of progressive destruction of periprosthetic bony tissue. Despite increased weight-bearing or increased mechanical load on a joint prosthesis, the literature does not support an increased rate of osteolysis or even an increase in radiological changes such as radiolucent lines or mal-alignment of the femoral or acetabular components postoperatively. The findings of Jackson and Lübbeke suggest that obesity is not associated with an increased rate of radiolucent lines. In the absence of these findings, this suggests that obesity does not pose an increased risk to the integrity of the implant. This was consistent across both cemented and uncemented implants [50, 51].

Revision surgery for THA is also found to be more common in obese patients, with revision rates of 8% reported in obese patients and 2.75% in non-obese patients [52, 53]. In obese patients who undergo revision surgery, re-infection rates and re-operation rates are higher than those who are not obese [54].

7.8 Super-Obesity

In this discussion, we have primarily classified patients as either obese or non-obese but have not considered the varying degrees of obesity. Super-obesity is a BMI >50. When compared with non-obese, obese, and morbidly obese patients, super-obese patients are found to have an increased risk of venous thromboembolism, infection, blood transfusion, and medical complications, along with dislocation readmission and revision [55]. In one study of 42 primary THA in super-obese patients, 24 had at least one complication either major or minor. Clinical outcomes and patient-reported outcomes in super-obese patients were much lower compared with other obesity subclasses. This would suggest that super-obesity is an independent risk factor in a patient considering THA [55–57].

7.9 Outcome Measures

The Harris Hip Score (HHS) is a clinician-based outcome measure and contains four subscales: pain, function, absence of deformity, and range of motion. It is used most commonly for the evaluation of outcomes post-THA. The Western Ontario and McMaster Universities Arthritis Index (WOMAC) was developed for use in osteoarthritis. WOMAC assesses patient-reported pain, stiffness, and physical function. Across a broad base of literature, HHS and WOMAC have been seen to improve in obese patients who undergo THA. Although research suggests the improvement in obese patients is lower compared with non-obese patients [58]. It has been found that patients undergoing total joint arthroplasty were more willing to proceed in lower-benefit higher-harm scenarios than surgeons. Further qualitative research is necessary to probe the obese patient's motivation and risk matrix in relation to THA [59].

7.10 Conclusion

As the evidence mounts for the improvement in function and range of movement throughout all BMI categories following THA, exclusion criteria for surgery for obese patients remain an area of ethical concern for many surgeons.

Many patients who are medically obese endure chronic pain and limited mobility daily due to their end-stage large joint osteoarthritis. While the role of THA in the treatment of these patients may require more consideration than in those who are not obese, many of these patients have such reduced quality of life that they still proceed to surgery despite understanding the increased risk in their perioperative period. Withholding 'the operation of the century' from what is projected to be over half the population by 2030 would not only be futile but would most likely reduce surgeon satisfaction, be anathema to equitable healthcare, and fail to ameliorate an orthopaedic subset of the public health crisis that is obesity. Our role as surgeons should be centred around how best to equitably select, optimise preoperatively, and perfect perioperatively the strategies, techniques, and components required to reduce the risks to patients—and surgical staff—for obese patients undergoing total hip arthroplasty.

References

1. Obesity and overweight [Internet]. [cited 2023 Feb 5]. Available from: https://www.who.int/news-room/fact-sheets/detail/obesity-and-overweight.
2. Wang Y, Beydoun MA, Liang L, Caballero B, Kumanyika SK. Will all Americans become overweight or obese? Estimating the progression and cost of the US obesity epidemic. Obesity (Silver Spring). 2008;16(10):2323–30.
3. Wang YC, McPherson K, Marsh T, Gortmaker SL, Brown M. Health and economic burden of the projected obesity trends in the USA and the UK. Lancet. 2011;378(9793):815–25.
4. Man G, Mologhianu G. Osteoarthritis pathogenesis—a complex process that involves the entire joint. J Med Life. 2014;7(1):37–41.
5. Guilak F. Biomechanical factors in osteoarthritis. Best Pract Res Clin Rheumatol. 2011;25(6):815–23.
6. Stürmer T, Günther KP, Brenner H. Obesity, overweight and patterns of osteoarthritis: the Ulm osteoarthritis study. J Clin Epidemiol. 2000;53(3):307–13.
7. Järvholm B, Lewold S, Malchau H, Vingård E. Age, bodyweight, smoking habits and the risk of severe osteoarthritis in the hip and knee in men. Eur J Epidemiol. 2005;20(6):537–42.
8. Carender CN, Glass NA, DeMik DE, Elkins JM, Brown TS, Bedard NA. Projected prevalence of obesity in primary total hip arthroplasty: how big will the problem get? J Arthroplast. 2022;37(5):874–9.
9. Flugsrud GB, Nordsletten L, Espehaug B, Havelin LI, Engeland A, Meyer HE. The impact of body mass index on later total hip arthroplasty for primary osteoarthritis: a cohort study in 1.2 million persons. Arthritis Rheum. 2006;54(3):802–7. https://doi.org/10.1002/art.21659.
10. Kunutsor SK, Whitehouse MR, Blom AW. Obesity paradox in joint replacement for osteoarthritis—truth or paradox? GeroScience. 2021;44(2):651–9.
11. Ma L, Yu X, Weng X, Lin J, Qian W, Huang Y. Obesity paradox among patients undergoing total knee arthroplasty: a retrospective cohort study. BMC Surg. 2022;22(1):373.
12. Valentijn TM, Galal W, Tjeertes EKM, Hoeks SE, Verhagen HJ, Stolker RJ. The obesity paradox in the surgical population. Surgeon. 2013;11(3):169–76.
13. Houdek MT, Griffin AM, Ferguson PC, Wunder JS. Morbid obesity increases the risk of postoperative wound complications, infection, and repeat surgical procedures following upper extremity limb salvage surgery for soft tissue sarcoma. Hand (N Y). 2019;14(1):114–20.
14. Dowsey MM, Choong PFM. Obesity is a major risk factor for prosthetic infection after primary hip arthroplasty. Clin Orthop Relat Res. 2008;466(1):153–8.
15. Jiang J, Teng Y, Fan Z, Khan S, Xia Y. Does obesity affect the surgical outcome and complication rates of spinal surgery? A meta-analysis. Clin Orthop Relat Res. 2014;472(3):968–75.
16. DeMik DE, Kohler JG, Carender CN, Glass NA, Brown TS, Bedard NA. What is the impact of body mass index cutoffs on total hip arthroplasty complications? J Arthroplast. 2022;37(7):1320–1325.e1.
17. Carender CN, DeMik DE, Elkins JM, Brown TS, Bedard NA. Are body mass index cutoffs creating racial, ethnic, and gender disparities in eligibility for primary total hip and knee arthroplasty? J Arthroplast. 2022;37(6):1009–16.
18. Changulani M, Kalairajah Y, Peel T, Field RE. The relationship between obesity and the age at which hip and knee replacement is undertaken. J Bone Joint Surg Br. 2008;90-B(3):360–3.
19. Maradit Kremers H, Visscher SL, Kremers WK, Naessens JM, Lewallen DG. Obesity increases length of stay and direct medical costs in total hip arthroplasty. Clin Orthop Relat Res. 2014;472(4):1232–9.

20. Smith NA, Martin G, Marginson B. Preoperative assessment and prehabilitation in patients with obesity undergoing non-bariatric surgery: a systematic review. J Clin Anesth. 2022;78:110676.
21. Smith TO, Aboelmagd T, Hing CB, MacGregor A. Does bariatric surgery prior to total hip or knee arthroplasty reduce post-operative complications and improve clinical outcomes for obese patients? Bone Joint J. 2016;98-B(9):1160–6.
22. Murr MM, Streiff WJ, Ndindjock R. A literature review and summary recommendations of the impact of bariatric surgery on orthopedic outcomes. Obes Surg. 2021;31(1):394–400.
23. Liu J, Zhong H, Poeran J, Sculco PK, Kim DH, Memtsoudis SG. Bariatric surgery and total knee/hip arthroplasty: an analysis of the impact of sequence and timing on outcomes. Reg Anesth Pain Med. 2021;46(11):941–5.
24. Bains SS, Sax OC, Chen Z, Nabet A, Nace J, Delanois RE. Bariatric surgery prior to total hip arthroplasty: does timing or type matter? Hip Int. 2023;33(6):1017–25.
25. Ryan SP, Couch CG, Duong SQ, Taunton MJ, Lewallen DG, Berry DJ, et al. Frank Stinchfield award: does bariatric surgery prior to primary total hip arthroplasty really improve outcomes? J Arthroplast. 2022;37(7S):S386–90.
26. Seward MW, Chen AF. Obesity, preoperative weight loss, and telemedicine before total joint arthroplasty: a review. Arthroplasty. 2022;4(1):2.
27. Bowditch MG, Villar RN. Do obese patients bleed more? A prospective study of blood loss at total hip replacement. Ann R Coll Surg Engl. 1999;81(3):198–200.
28. Dienstknecht T, Lüring C, Tingart M, Grifka J, Sendtner E. A minimally invasive approach for total hip arthroplasty does not diminish early post-operative outcome in obese patients: a prospective, randomised trial. Int Orthop. 2013;37(6):1013–8.
29. Elson LC, Barr CJ, Chandran SE, Hansen VJ, Malchau H, Kwon YM. Are morbidly obese patients undergoing total hip arthroplasty at an increased risk for component malpositioning? J Arthroplast. 2013;28(8, Suppl):41–4.
30. Lester JD, Hsu S, Ahmad CS. Occupational hazards facing orthopedic surgeons. Am J Orthop (Belle Mead NJ). 2012;41(3):132–9.
31. AlQahtani SM, Alzahrani MM, Harvey EJ. Prevalence of musculoskeletal disorders among orthopedic trauma surgeons: an OTA survey. Can J Surg. 2016;59(1):42–7.
32. Alqahtani SM, Alzahrani MM, Tanzer M. Adult reconstructive surgery: a high-risk profession for work-related injuries. J Arthroplast. 2016;31(6):1194–8.
33. McQuivey KS, Christopher ZK, Deckey DG, Mi L, Bingham JS, Spangehl MJ. Surgical ergonomics and musculoskeletal pain in arthroplasty surgeons. J Arthroplast. 2021;36(11):3781–7.e7.
34. Khan IA, Haffar A, Magnuson JA, Ong C, Austin MS, Krueger CA, et al. Surgeons experience greater cardiorespiratory strain and stress during total hip arthroplasty than total knee arthroplasty. J Arthroplast. 2022;37(4):637–41.
35. Haynes J, Nam D, Barrack RL. Obesity in total hip arthroplasty: does it make a difference? Bone Joint J. 2017;99-B(1_Suppl_A):31–6.
36. Motaghedi R, Bae JJ, Memtsoudis SG, Kim DH, Beathe JC, Paroli L, et al. Association of obesity with inflammation and pain after total hip arthroplasty. Clin Orthop Relat Res. 2014;472(5):1442–8.
37. Thelwall S, Harrington P, Sheridan E, Lamagni T. Impact of obesity on the risk of wound infection following surgery: results from a nationwide prospective multicentre cohort study in England. Clin Microbiol Infect. 2015;21(11):1008.e1–8.
38. McCalden RW, Charron KD, MacDonald SJ, Bourne RB, Naudie DD. Does morbid obesity affect the outcome of total hip replacement?: an analysis of 3290 THRs. J Bone Joint Surg Br. 2011;93(3):321–5.
39. Haverkamp D, Klinkenbijl MN, Somford MP, Albers GHR, van der Vis HM. Obesity in total hip arthroplasty—does it really matter? Acta Orthop. 2011;82(4):417–22.
40. Janson B, Thursky K. Dosing of antibiotics in obesity. Curr Opin Infect Dis. 2012;25(6):634–49.
41. Watts CD, Houdek MT, Wagner ER, Sculco PK, Chalmers BP, Taunton MJ. High risk of wound complications following direct anterior total hip arthroplasty in obese patients. J Arthroplast. 2015;30(12):2296–8.

42. Shah NV, Huddleston HP, Wolff DT, Newman JM, Pivec R, Naziri Q, et al. Does surgical approach for total hip arthroplasty impact infection risk in the obese patient? A systematic review. Orthopedics. 2022;45(2):e67–72.
43. Purcell RL, Parks NL, Gargiulo JM, Hamilton WG. Severely obese patients have a higher risk of infection after direct anterior approach total hip arthroplasty. J Arthroplast. 2016;31(9 Suppl):162–5.
44. Russo MW, Macdonell JR, Paulus MC, Keller JM, Zawadsky MW. Increased complications in obese patients undergoing direct anterior total hip arthroplasty. J Arthroplast. 2015;30(8):1384–7.
45. Zhang J, Wyatt MC, Frampton CM, Anderson G. Does surgical approach affect early outcomes following primary total hip replacement in obese patients? Hip Int. 2021;31(3):304–10.
46. Rhind JH, Baker C, Roberts PJ. Total hip arthroplasty in the obese patient: tips and tricks and review of the literature. Indian J Orthop. 2020;54(6):776–83.
47. Maisongrosse P, Lepage B, Cavaignac E, Pailhe R, Reina N, Chiron P, et al. Obesity is no longer a risk factor for dislocation after total hip arthroplasty with a double-mobility cup. Int Orthop. 2015;39(7):1251–8.
48. Fessy MH, Jacquot L, Rollier JC, Chouteau J, Ait-Si-Selmi T, Bothorel H, et al. Midterm clinical and radiographic outcomes of a contemporary monoblock dual-mobility cup in uncemented total hip arthroplasty. J Arthroplast. 2019;34(12):2983–91.
49. Azodi OS, Adami J, Lindström D, Eriksson KO, Wladis A, Bellocco R. High body mass index is associated with increased risk of implant dislocation following primary total hip replacement: 2,106 patients followed for up to 8 years. Acta Orthop. 2008;79(1):141–7.
50. Jackson MP, Sexton SA, Yeung E, Walter WL, Walter WK, Zicat BA. The effect of obesity on the mid-term survival and clinical outcome of cementless total hip replacement. J Bone Joint Surg. 2009;91-B(10):1296–300.
51. Lübbeke A, Garavaglia G, Barea C, Roussos C, Stern R, Hoffmeyer P. Influence of obesity on femoral osteolysis five and ten years following total hip arthroplasty. JBJS. 2010;92(10):1964.
52. Barrett M, Prasad A, Boyce L, Dawson-Bowling S, Achan P, Millington S, et al. Total hip arthroplasty outcomes in morbidly obese patients: a systematic review. EFORT Open Rev. 2018;3(9):507–12.
53. McLaughlin JR, Lee KR. The outcome of total hip replacement in obese and non-obese patients at 10- to 18-years. J Bone Joint Surg Br. 2006;88-B(10):1286–92.
54. Pulos N, McGraw MH, Courtney PM, Lee GC. Revision THA in obese patients is associated with high re-operation rates at short-term follow-up. J Arthroplast. 2014;29(9, Suppl):209–13.
55. Werner BC, Higgins MD, Pehlivan HC, Carothers JT, Browne JA. Super obesity is an independent risk factor for complications after primary total hip arthroplasty. J Arthroplast. 2017;32(2):402–6.
56. Arsoy D, Woodcock JA, Lewallen DG, Trousdale RT. Outcomes and complications following total hip arthroplasty in the super-obese patient, BMI > 50. J Arthroplast. 2014;29(10):1899–905.
57. Rajgopal R, Martin R, Howard JL, Somerville L, MacDonald SJ, Bourne R. Outcomes and complications of total hip replacement in super-obese patients. Bone Joint J. 2013;95-B(6):758–63.
58. Jameson SS, Mason JM, Baker PN, Elson DW, Deehan DJ, Reed MR. The impact of body mass index on patient reported outcome measures (PROMs) and complications following primary hip arthroplasty. J Arthroplast. 2014;29(10):1889–98.
59. Fontana MA, Medina CK, Kohilakis EC, Pearle AD, MacLean CH, McLawhorn AS. Patient and surgeon risk-taking regarding total joint arthroplasty. J Arthroplast. 2022;37(4):624–9.e18.

Obesity and Knee Disorders

8

John Scanlon, Matthew Macciacchera, and Adrian Cassar-Gheiti

8.1 The Knee

The knee is a modified hinge joint and functions to support an individual's body weight and allow for efficient and stable walking. The bony components of the knee consist of the femur, tibia, and patella. The femoral condyles articulate with the tibial plateau to form the tibiofemoral joint and the patella articulates with the trochlear groove of the femur to form the patellofemoral joint. The femoral condyles are 8–9° valgus to the anatomical axis, whereas the tibial plateau is 2–3° varus to the anatomical axis. The bony components and muscles of the knee function as a third-class lever system to allow for flexion and extension as well as a lesser degree of internal and external rotation.

The four primary ligaments that stabilise the knee are the anterior cruciate, posterior cruciate, medial collateral, and lateral collateral ligaments. These ligaments function to resist anterior and posterior tibial translation, and valgus and varus stresses, respectively. The menisci are crescent-shaped tissues located on the medial and lateral aspects of the knee joint [1]. The menisci function to act as shock absorbers, distribute load, and provide stability to the knee joint [1]. The articular surfaces of the knee are lined by cartilage, which functions to minimise friction and dissipate forces through the knee joint [2].

Obesity is a modifiable risk factor that results in increased joint stress and load forces on the knee, which, in turn, can predispose patients to the development of knee pathologies such as osteoarthritis, soft-tissue injuries, as well as result in an increased risk and severity of traumatic bony injuries [3].

J. Scanlon (✉) · M. Macciacchera
Royal College of Surgeons in Ireland, Dublin, Ireland
e-mail: scanlojo@tcd.ie; matthewmacciacchera@rcsi.ie

A. Cassar-Gheiti
National Orthopaedic Hospital Cappagh, Dublin, Ireland

J. M. O´Byrne et al. (eds.), *Musculoskeletal Disease and Obesity*,
https://doi.org/10.1007/978-3-031-63310-2_8

8.2 Meniscal Tears

Obesity is a risk factor for meniscal injury, and obese patients with meniscal injuries experience a greater loss of knee function and worse knee pain than non-obese individuals [4, 5].

8.2.1 Pathophysiology

An increase in torque acting on the knee during rotational movements places obese individuals at an increased risk of meniscal injury. A diminished vascular supply secondary to obesity-related comorbidities can impair healing.

8.2.2 Management

The initial management of suspected meniscal tears in obese and non-obese patients alike should consist of RICE with analgesia for 4–6 weeks. The majority of meniscal injuries will resolve with conservative management.

Obesity increases the risk of patients requiring operative management, and morbidly obese individuals are at a 15–25-fold increased risk of meniscus injuries requiring surgery [4]. Operative management includes meniscal repair, and partial and complete meniscectomy. Meniscal repair is preferred to meniscectomy, when possible, to prevent the development of osteoarthritis, particularly in obese individuals.

8.2.3 Outcomes

For those that require surgical management, there is significant improvement in symptoms; however, the postoperative levels of pain and knee function are inferior to non-obese patients [5]. There is no evidence to suggest that obese individuals have a higher complication or failure rate following meniscal surgery [6].

8.3 Tibial Plateau Fracture

Tibial plateau fractures are periarticular injuries of the proximal tibia frequently associated with soft-tissue injuries. The severity of a tibial plateau fracture and the complexity of its treatment depend on the force imparted to the affected knee. Obesity has some protective effects in reducing fracture risk such as increased bone mineral density and a 'cushion effect' from extra adipose tissue [7, 8]. However, the increased force overpowers the protective effects and results in an increased fracture risk and an increased fracture severity in an obese population [9, 10].

Table 8.1 Shatzker Classification

Type 1	Wedge-shaped pure cleavage fracture of the lateral tibial plateau
Type 2	Splitting and depression of the lateral tibial plateau
Type 3	Pure depression of the lateral tibial plateau
Type 4	Medial tibial plateau fracture with a split or depressed component
Type 5	Wedge fracture of both lateral and medial tibial plateau
Type 6	Transverse tibial metadiaphyseal fracture with any type of tibial plateau fracture

8.3.1 Fracture Patterns

Tibial plateau fractures are commonly classified according to the Schatzker classification system (Table 8.1) [11]. The most common fracture locations are the lateral plateau, followed by bicondylar and medial plateau. Types 4–6 are high-energy injuries associated with joint instability from subluxation to dislocation.

Obese patients are more likely to have bicondylar or type 5 tibial plateau fractures [10]. Tibial plateau fractures involving the medial tibial plateau carry an increased risk of several soft-tissue complications, including medial meniscus tears, anterior cruciate ligament (ACL) injuries, and compartment syndrome [12, 13].

8.3.2 Management

Low-energy minimally displaced tibial plateau fractures may be managed with non-operative measures such as weight-bearing restrictions and the use of a hinged-knee brace.

As high-energy fracture patterns are common in the obese population, operative management is commonly required. Operative management options for tibial plateau fractures include acute open reduction internal fixation commonly with screw-plate constructs. Alternatively, external fixators can be used as either staged or definitive options in cases with severe soft-tissue injury or severely comminuted fractures that are not amenable to fixation.

8.3.3 Postoperative Challenges

The risk of a surgical complication increases by approximately 4% per increase in BMI point in the obese population [10]. Obese patients are at an increased risk of deep surgical-site infections, wound dehiscence, and venous thromboembolism [10].

8.4 Ultralow-Velocity Knee Dislocation

Knee dislocations are uncommon but are a potentially limb-threatening injury due to frequent concurrent neurovascular injury. Knee dislocations are usually the result of high-energy trauma; however, for the morbidly obese population

(BMI > 40), the term 'ultralow velocity' knee dislocation has been coined to describe patients who sustain knee dislocations secondary to low-energy injuries such as falls from standing height or even spontaneous knee dislocations on standing [14, 15].

8.4.1 Pathoanatomy

Knee dislocations are typically characterised by multiligamentous injury in which at least two primary knee ligaments are injured. Associated neurovascular injury is common, and rates of up to 48% have been reported following knee dislocation in morbidly obese patients [14, 16].

8.4.2 Diagnosis

Ultralow velocity knee dislocation is an orthopaedic emergency must be recognised early. A low-velocity mechanism of injury and a deformity that may be concealed by a high BMI can lead to missed diagnoses. Knee dislocation may be apparent on radiographs; however, as spontaneous reduction is common, the knee ligaments should be carefully assessed [17]. Stress view X-rays may be helpful in cases where ligamentous assessment is limited by a high BMI.

8.4.3 Management

Knee dislocation should be reduced emergently either under sedation or in theatre. Absolute indications for surgery are irreducible dislocations, open dislocations, and vascular injury [18]. Persistent instability may be controlled with the use of an external fixator or hinge knee brace. Following reduction, arthroscopy with ACL or PCL reconstruction is generally required.

8.4.4 Outcomes

Ligamentous reconstruction following ultralow velocity knee dislocation results in improved outcomes compared to conservative management; however, there are high rates of morbidity and patient satisfaction is poor [14, 16]. Postoperative complications are common and include surgical-site infection, arthrofibrosis, arthritis, persistent instability, venous thromboembolism, claudication, above-knee amputation, and death [14, 16].

8.5 Anterior Knee Pain

Anterior knee pain is a common knee condition in young patients characterised by peripatellar or retropatellar pain that often occurs during activities that burden the patellofemoral joint, such as using stairs, squatting, kneeling, or jumping [19]. During these activities, the force of an individual's body weight across the joint may be multiplied by up to a factor of 5, as such patients with anterior knee pain are more likely to be obese [20].

8.5.1 Aetiology

There are multiple causes of anterior knee pain, each of which may present in a similar manner. The causes include osteoarthritis of the patellofemoral joint, patellar tendinopathy, overuse injuries, traumatic events, and malignment. Given the large overlap in possible presentations, meticulous history-taking and exams are important in determining a diagnosis.

8.5.2 Outcomes

Obese individuals with patellofemoral pain are more likely to have a reduced functional capacity [21]. The interventional outcomes for obese patients are similar to a non-obese cohort [20]. Importantly, patients with patellofemoral pain are more likely to develop osteoarthritis later in life [22].

8.6 Osteoarthritis

Osteoarthritis is a degenerative joint disease affecting the articular cartilage which has a relative inability to heal due to its avascular and hypocellular nature [23]. The increased prevalence of obesity has led to an increase in knee osteoarthritis and subsequently an increase in the demand for total knee arthroplasty (TKA) [24]. TKA results in a significant symptomatic relief from osteoarthritis for patients regardless of BMI; however, there are associated challenges for the surgeon to consider when performing arthroplasty for an obese patient [25].

8.6.1 Pathophysiology

Obesity results in accelerated cartilage degeneration and early osteoarthritis due to increased mechanical forces exerted on the joint. Metabolic mechanisms contribute as adipose tissue secretes pro-inflammatory cytokines and adipocytokines that produce a catabolic effect and alter the homeostasis of cartilage [26, 27]. As such, obese patients are more likely to develop arthritis in non-load-bearing joints, such as the hand, as well as load-bearing joints [27, 28].

8.6.2 TKA Postoperative Challenges

Morbid obesity results in increased rates of complications following total knee arthroplasty [29]. Obese patients are at an increased risk of developing infection and requiring revision [25, 29]. The most common reasons for revision following TKA are infection, followed by aseptic loosening and periprosthetic fracture [30]. Higher implant–bone stress levels contribute to increased rates of aseptic loosening in obese patients [31]. The tibial component is at particular risk in this cohort, and a stemmed tibial component should be considered to reduce the need for revision due to aseptic loosening [32].

Factors that may contribute to an increased complication rate include comorbidities such as a weakened immune response, and an increased operating time secondary to a more technically demanding surgery and larger wounds requiring a longer closure time [33].

8.6.3 Benefits

There are challenges encountered in performing a TKA for an obese patient; however, the postoperative improvements in knee function and quality of life are similar to non-obese patients [25]. Despite an increase in functional outcomes, TKA results in weight loss for only approximately 7% of obese patients [34]. The majority of obese patients who require TKA have no change or an increase in BMI postoperatively [34, 35].

8.7 Summary

Obesity is becoming increasingly common and is associated with more severe injury from low-velocity trauma. Obesity can limit clinical assessment of knee injuries, cause challenges in the surgical management of knee injuries, and can predispose patients to complications and inferior outcomes following management.

References

1. Fox AJ, Bedi A, Rodeo SA. The basic science of human knee menisci: structure, composition, and function. Sports Health. 2012;4(4):340–51.
2. Gomoll AH, Minas T. The quality of healing: articular cartilage. Wound Repair Regen. 2014;22(Suppl 1):30–8.
3. Singer SP, Dammerer D, Krismer M, Liebensteiner MC. Maximum lifetime body mass index is the appropriate predictor of knee and hip osteoarthritis. Arch Orthop Trauma Surg. 2018;138(1):99–103.
4. Ford GM, Hegmann KT, White GL Jr, Holmes EB. Associations of body mass index with meniscal tears. Am J Prev Med. 2005;28(4):364–8.
5. Zhang T, Jauregui JJ, Foster M, Packer JD, Meredith SJ, Leong NL, et al. Outcomes of partial meniscectomy in obese patients: a systematic review and meta-analysis. Cartilage. 2020;13(1_suppl):216S–27S.
6. Sommerfeldt MF, Magnussen RA, Randall KL, Tompkins M, Perkins B, Sharma A, et al. The relationship between body mass index and risk of failure following meniscus repair. J Knee Surg. 2016;29(8):645–8.
7. Ishii S, Cauley JA, Greendale GA, Nielsen C, Karvonen-Gutierrez C, Ruppert K, et al. Pleiotropic effects of obesity on fracture risk: the study of women's health across the nation. J Bone Miner Res. 2014;29(12):2561–70.
8. Arbabi S, Wahl WL, Hemmila MR, Kohoyda-Inglis C, Taheri PA, Wang SC. The cushion effect. J Trauma. 2003;54(6):1090–3.
9. Parratte S, Pesenti S, Argenson JN. Obesity in orthopedics and trauma surgery. Orthop Traumatol Surg Res. 2014;100(1 Suppl):S91–7.
10. McGurk KM, Traven SA, McCadden A, LeBrun CT, Reid KR, Hartsock LA, et al. Elevated body mass index is associated with tibial plateau fracture complexity and post-operative complications. Trauma. 2022;25(3):214–21.
11. Schatzker J, McBroom R, Bruce D. The tibial plateau fracture. The Toronto experience 1968–1975. Clin Orthop Relat Res. 1979;138:94–104.
12. Stark E, Stucken C, Trainer G, Tornetta PI. Compartment syndrome in Schatzker type VI plateau fractures and medial condylar fracture-dislocations treated with temporary external fixation. J Orthop Trauma. 2009;23(7):502–6.
13. Stannard JP, Lopez R, Volgas D. Soft tissue injury of the knee after tibial plateau fractures. J Knee Surg. 2010;23(4):187–92.
14. Azar FM, Brandt JC, Miller RH 3rd, Phillips BB. Ultra-low-velocity knee dislocations. Am J Sports Med. 2011;39(10):2170–4.
15. Hagino RT, DeCaprio JD, Valentine RJ, Clagett GP. Spontaneous popliteal vascular injury in the morbidly obese. J Vasc Surg. 1998;28(3):458–62. discussion 62–3
16. Werner BC, Gwathmey FW Jr, Higgins ST, Hart JM, Miller MD. Ultra-low velocity knee dislocations: patient characteristics, complications, and outcomes. Am J Sports Med. 2014;42(2):358–63.
17. Wascher DC, Dvirnak PC, DeCoster TA. Knee dislocation: initial assessment and implications for treatment. J Orthop Trauma. 1997;11(7):525–9.
18. Levy BA, Fanelli GC, Whelan DB, Stannard JP, MacDonald PA, Boyd JL, et al. Controversies in the treatment of knee dislocations and multiligament reconstruction. J Am Acad Orthop Surg. 2009;17(4):197–206.
19. Reilly DT, Martens M. Experimental analysis of the quadriceps muscle force and patello-femoral joint reaction force for various activities. Acta Orthop Scand. 1972;43(2):126–37.
20. Hart HF, Barton CJ, Khan KM, Riel H, Crossley KM. Is body mass index associated with patellofemoral pain and patellofemoral osteoarthritis? A systematic review and meta-regression and analysis. Br J Sports Med. 2017;51(10):781–90.

21. Ferreira AS, Mentiplay BF, Taborda B, Pazzinatto MF, de Azevedo FM, de Oliveira SD. Overweight and obesity in young adults with patellofemoral pain: impact on functional capacity and strength. J Sport Health Sci. 2023;12(2):202–11.
22. Thomas MJ, Wood L, Selfe J, Peat G. Anterior knee pain in younger adults as a precursor to subsequent patellofemoral osteoarthritis: a systematic review. BMC Musculoskelet Disord. 2010;11(1):201.
23. Ambra LF, Franciozi CE, Phan A, Faloppa F, Gomoll AH. Isolated MPTL reconstruction fails to restore lateral patellar stability when compared to MPFL reconstruction. Knee Surg Sports Traumatol Arthrosc. 2021;29(3):793–9.
24. Powell A, Teichtahl AJ, Wluka AE, Cicuttini FM. Obesity: a preventable risk factor for large joint osteoarthritis which may act through biomechanical factors. Br J Sports Med. 2005;39(1):4–5.
25. Boyce L, Prasad A, Barrett M, Dawson-Bowling S, Millington S, Hanna SA, et al. The outcomes of total knee arthroplasty in morbidly obese patients: a systematic review of the literature. Arch Orthop Trauma Surg. 2019;139(4):553–60.
26. Sowers MR, Karvonen-Gutierrez CA. The evolving role of obesity in knee osteoarthritis. Curr Opin Rheumatol. 2010;22(5):533–7.
27. Pottie P, Presle N, Terlain B, Netter P, Mainard D, Berenbaum F. Obesity and osteoarthritis: more complex than predicted! Ann Rheum Dis. 2006;65(11):1403–5.
28. Grotle M, Hagen KB, Natvig B, Dahl FA, Kvien TK. Obesity and osteoarthritis in knee, hip and/or hand: an epidemiological study in the general population with 10 years follow-up. BMC Musculoskelet Disord. 2008;9:132.
29. Malinzak RA, Ritter MA, Berend ME, Meding JB, Olberding EM, Davis KE. Morbidly obese, diabetic, younger, and unilateral joint arthroplasty patients have elevated total joint arthroplasty infection rates. J Arthroplast. 2009;24(6 Suppl):84–8.
30. Postler A, Lützner C, Beyer F, Tille E, Lützner J. Analysis of total knee arthroplasty revision causes. BMC Musculoskelet Disord. 2018;19(1):55.
31. Bourne RB, Finlay JB. The influence of tibial component intramedullary stems and implant-cortex contact on the strain distribution of the proximal tibia following total knee arthroplasty. An in vitro study. Clin Orthop Relat Res. 1986;208:95–9.
32. Schultz BJ, DeBaun MR, Huddleston JI 3rd. The use of stems for morbid obesity in total knee arthroplasty. J Knee Surg. 2019;32(7):607–10.
33. Gadinsky NE, Manuel JB, Lyman S, Westrich GH. Increased operating room time in patients with obesity during primary total knee arthroplasty: conflicts for scheduling. J Arthroplast. 2012;27(6):1171–6.
34. Coelho A, Leal-Blanquet J, Sánchez-Soler J, Torres-Claramunt R, Hinarejos P, Monllau J. Patients lose weight after a total knee arthroplasty: myth or reality? Int Orthop. 2022;46(6):1299–304.
35. Riddle DL, Singh JA, Harmsen WS, Schleck CD, Lewallen DG. Clinically important body weight gain following knee arthroplasty: a five-year comparative cohort study. Arthritis Care Res (Hoboken). 2013;65(5):669–77.

9 Obesity and Foot and Ankle Disorders

Lyndon Y. H. Low, Nuala McAuley, and Adeel Memon

9.1 Introduction

Obesity is a world epidemic and has become one of the major public health problems in modern society. Its association with increased risk for diabetes, hypertension, and other cardiovascular diseases, as well as for certain musculoskeletal disorders, especially hip and knee osteoarthritis, is very well studied. However, the foot and ankle are not immune to the effects of obesity. Foot pain is also a common complaint amongst adults with a raised body mass index (BMI), where it is prevalent in 40% of obese patients compared to 11% in patients with normal weights. Increased body mass is associated with poor foot function as this alters gait and increases biomechanical loads, in addition to the metabolic effects of excess adipose tissue [1].

9.2 Normal Foot and Ankle Biomechanics

Foot and ankle problems in the obese population are thought to be secondary to the extra mechanical stress of carrying additional weight [2]. To understand how obesity affects the foot and ankle, it is first important to understand the three rockers of normal gait [3]. The gait cycle ranges from one heel-strike to the next heel-strike of the ipsilateral leg and comprises two phases: the stance phase and the swing phase. The stance phase makes up 65% of the gait cycle which extends from heel-strike to toe-off on the same foot, while the swing phase makes up the remaining 35% from

L. Y. H. Low (✉) · N. McAuley
Royal College of Surgeons Ireland, Dublin 2, Ireland
e-mail: lowl@tcd.ie

A. Memon
Mater Private Network Cork, Cork, Ireland
e-mail: adeel.memon@materprivate.ie

J. M. O´Byrne et al. (eds.), *Musculoskeletal Disease and Obesity*,
https://doi.org/10.1007/978-3-031-63310-2_9

toe-off to heel-strike once again on the same foot. The first two rockers are thought to be deceleration rockers involving eccentric muscle contraction, consisting of the active lengthening of the muscle fibres. The third rocker is an acceleration rocker, hence concentrically contracts, resulting in the active shortening of muscle fibres [4, 5].

The first (heel) rocker is involved when the landing foot prepares to receive the load. The heel briefly exerts a contact force with the ground with an equal but opposite ground reaction force. This is the short period between heel-strike and foot-flat phase of the gait cycle. As the ground reaction force is posterior to the ankle joint, the ankle now moves from neutral to 10 degrees of plantarflexion and internal rotation, controlled carefully by the eccentric contraction of the tibialis anterior. The foot acts as a shock absorber, although at relatively lower loads due to dual-limb support in the first rocker [5, 6].

The second (ankle) rocker is when the foot is firmly planted onto the ground, allowing the supporting leg and the rest of the body to move forwards. This is a longer period between foot-flat and toe-off and is also a dynamic phase where that 10-degree ankle plantarflexion changes to 10 degrees of ankle dorsiflexion and external rotation. This is due to the arc motion of the leg relative to the foot as the centre of gravity of the body moves forward relative to the ankle joint, that is, the ground reaction force vector moving anterior to the ankle. The rate of dorsiflexion is controlled by the eccentric contraction of the gastrocnemius and soleus. The foot remains flexible and soft to absorb energy via a single limb, made possible by eversion of the subtalar joint so that the transverse tarsal joints are parallel to each other [5]. The foot pronates with flattening of the arch to adapt to the surface [6].

Lastly, the third (forefoot) rocker takes place in the forefoot in the time frame between heel-off and toe-off. The ankle plantarflexors contract concentrically to produce ankle plantarflexion as the heel rises, and the toes progressively extend until toe-off occurs. The foot changes into a rigid lever arm by inversion of the subtalar joint to rotate the transverse tarsal joints into an incongruent alignment. The plantar fascia also tightens with toe extension, raising the foot arch and contributing to the rigidity of the foot as a lever. The latter is the 'Windlass' effect, and these allow for the forward propulsion of the body [5].

9.3 Obesity and Altered Biomechanics

Obesity is also associated with decreased gait speed, a shorter stride length, prolonged double support time in walking, and an increased overall stance time [7, 8], thereby peak pressure across the midfoot. During the gait cycle, obese individuals take significantly wider step widths, a predominance of ankle dorsiflexion in the gait cycle, and a diminution of ankle plantarflexion [8]. Reduced plantarflexion during terminal stance can be explained by possible weakness in the plantarflexors of obese individuals. As these muscles are partial contributors to ankle joint moments in the sagittal plane, the push-off ability is decreased [9]. In an attempt to increase stability and accommodate for a large thigh circumference, step width is contributed by decreased Q angles and hip abduction angles, while the foot is abducted with an earlier flat-foot occurrence in the stance phase of gait [2, 8]. Obese individuals were found to spend approximately 2.5% longer in the stance phase, 5% longer in double support, and 2% less time in single support than their non-obese counterparts [1, 10].

9.4 Non-Specific Foot Pain

The foot serves as the primary region in the body responsible for regulating the forces generated by ground contact. This area experiences both bending and torsional loads, impacting both the bones and soft tissues [11]. Previous studies have demonstrated associations between obesity and foot pain [1, 12, 13]. The underlying mechanism is nevertheless poorly understood in general [14], but are thought to be biomechanical and metabolic. Obese individuals have flatter and larger feet, reduced range of motion, and generate larger forces across the plantar as surfaces of their foot during the gait cycle, leading to excessive loads exerted on osseous and soft-tissue structures [15]. From a functional perspective, Mickle and Steel [1] have shown that obese individuals have weaker toe flexor muscles and intrinsic foot muscles such as the flexor hallucis brevis, flexor digitorum brevis, and abductor hallucis. These are key contributors to the medial longitudinal arch and hence a resultant lowered arch in the obese population [16]. There is a relationship between high peak plantar pressures and foot pain, which, in the context of obesity and the constant need to bear excessive mass, is explained by excess stress/strain on the structures of the foot [15, 17]. Butterworth et al. found that the greatest predictor of plantar force and pressure throughout the forefoot, midfoot, and hindfoot was bodyweight [15]. Wearing et al. alternatively suggested that fat mass under the midfoot, rather than structural foot changes, is the cause of increased midfoot plantar pressures [18].

From a metabolic standpoint, the development of foot pain is proposed to be secondary to excess adipose tissue and its dysregulation in obesity. There is a downregulation of beneficial adipokines and an overproduction of proinflammatory cytokines [13], the latter of which has been shown to be associated with hyperalgesia and progression to chronic pain [19]. Avoidance of pain leads to further alterations in normal gait pattern and creates a vicious cycle.

9.5 Plantar Fasciitis

Increased BMI is also strongly associated with chronic plantar heel pain, of which its primary cause is plantar fasciitis [12, 20] in the obese population. However, the causality is uncertain as it is also possible that obesity develops as a result of decreased physical activity secondary to chronic plantar heel pain [12]. Riddle et al. also found that individuals with a BMI >30 kg/m^2 are also at increased risk for the development of plantar fasciitis, with an odds ratio of 5.6 compared to those with a BMI ≤25 [20]. Although the increased mechanical load from a higher BMI is a probable source of plantar fasciitis, incident and prevalent foot pain is found to be more strongly associated with fat mass compared to fat-free mass, suggesting that the adiposity-related inflammatory mechanisms are contributory to this condition [21].

It has also been demonstrated that an increased BMI causes a decrease in the stiffness of plantar fascia, increased thickness of the plantar fascia, and a thicker heel pad [22]. The architectural and mechanical changes in the heel pad and plantar fascia lead to a diminished cushioning and supportive capacity of the tissue in the role of supporting a rigid arch architecture [22, 23]. The increased heel pad thickness is considered a biological response to repetitive high-impact force caused by a raised BMI, but paradoxically does not increase shock absorbency [24]. The knock-on effects of decreased plantar fascia stiffness also extend to increase stress placed on the central metatarsals, plantar ligaments, and dorsal calcaneocuboid joints, which can cause fatigue failure and midfoot pain [22, 25].

9.6 Tendon Dysfunction and Pes Planus

The literature has suggested that individuals with tendon abnormalities, pain, rupture, or failure to respond to conservative management have significantly higher adiposity levels [26]. Load-bearing tendons are most frequently involved. Frey and Zamora in 2007 looked at the effects of obesity and being overweight on orthopaedic foot and ankle pathology in 1411 patients. They have demonstrated that patients with a BMI >25 were twice as likely to have tendinitis within the foot and ankle based on logistic regression, while plantar fasciitis and osteoarthritis were at an increased likelihood but not clinically significant. The cause of this is proposed to be secondary to overuse and increased stress on these structures due to increased body weight [2]. Weil et al. also found that patients with a higher BMI were linked to a higher incidence of Achilles tendinopathy, plantar fasciitis, and tibialis posterior tendinitis, as well as a lower success rate with conservative treatment of the above [27].

The recurring theme of the proposed mechanisms leading to tendinopathy includes increased strain on weight-bearing tendons and the biochemical changes caused by metabolic abnormalities. As obese individuals have more weight to bear, their weight-bearing tendons are exposed to greater loads, which can result in overuse tendinopathy [28]. Furthermore, adipose tissue is now recognised as an important signalling organ that releases several hormones and bioactive peptides, known as the adipokinome. These proteins, including chemerin, lipocalin 2, serum amyloid A3, leptin, and adiponectin, have various effects on mesenchymal cell phenotypes that can directly impact tendon structure. Adipokines have the ability to regulate the production of cytokines, prostanoids, and metalloproteinases. Obesity is associated with persistently raised serum levels of PGE2, TNF-α, and LTB4, indicating the presence of chronic, low-grade inflammation that may disrupt tendon homeostasis over an extended period [28, 29].

Pes planus is known to be a pain generator in the feet and lower legs [30]. Pes planus is more prevalent among children with overweight or obesity which has been reported to be up to 28%. It is not known whether carrying excess weight may be a cause of pes planus in children; studies have questioned whether pes planus may occur as a result of a lowered medial longitudinal arch after full development [30, 31] or a thicker midfoot plantar fat pad. A structural collapse can develop into a potentially disabling problem in later life as proper mechanics of the longitudinal arch are critical to normal foot function [31]. It can be hypothesised that in pes planus there is a greater preference for medial weight-bearing, leading to an altered lower extremity alignment [30] and increased mechanical strain on the medial longitudinal arch. When the capsuloligamentous structures, that is, static stabilisers become compromised, the tibialis posterior tendon and plantar fascia may become strained and symptomatic [32].

Furthermore, obese individuals tend to exhibit increased pronation of the foot. Irving et al. conducted a case-control study of 160 patients with and without chronic plantar heel pain, where they discovered symptomatic patients were more likely to be obese and have a pronated foot posture [33].

9.7 Obesity and Ankle Arthroplasty

In relation to arthroplasty and obesity, contemporary orthopaedic data suggests an increased incidence of revision, infection, decreased functional outcomes, and implant survival. However, the correlation between obesity and total ankle replacement on outcomes and complication rates is not well understood due to a paucity in the literature [34, 35] compared to the hip and knee arthroplasty counterparts. The incidence of complications requiring revision surgery in obese patients undergoing total ankle replacement was found to be around 18% [35]. Gross et al., in their study of 455 primary total ankle arthroplasty patients with a minimum of 2-year follow-up, found that obese patients experienced significant pain and functional improvements, however, with a lower functional outcome score than the control group [34]. Schipper et al., on the other hand, noted an increased long-term risk of implant failure among obese patients that was not seen in the intermediate term. Lastly, Werner et al. found that, in their study of 23,000 patients treated for end-stage ankle arthritis either with arthroplasty or arthrodesis, obese patients were linked to an increased risk of major and minor complications at 90 days, including infection, DVT, and incidence of revision surgery. Additionally, revision surgeries pose an additional risk to these individuals as the soft-tissue envelope is already threatened, further dissection or damage during revision surgery could lead to wound complications. Furthermore, one has to consider the bone loss during implant removal as the talus is devoid of reserve bone stock after the primary total ankle arthroplasty. Implant wear or loosening is a further concern in overweight individuals who undergo ankle arthroplasty as the implant may experience accelerated wear and tear [36].

References

1. Mickle KJ, Steele JR. Obese older adults suffer foot pain and foot-related functional limitation. Gait Posture. 2015;42(4):442–7.
2. Frey C, Zamora J. The effects of obesity on orthopaedic foot and ankle pathology. Foot Ankle Int. 2007;28(9):996–9.
3. Analysis G. Normal and pathological function. J Sports Sci Med. 2010;9(2):353.
4. Roig M, O'Brien K, Kirk G, Murray R, McKinnon P, Shadgan B, et al. The effects of eccentric versus concentric resistance training on muscle strength and mass in healthy adults: a systematic review with meta-analysis. Br J Sports Med. 2009;43(8):556–68.
5. Malik SS, Malik SS. Biomechanics of the ankle and foot. In: Orthopaedic biomechanics made easy. Cambridge: Cambridge University Press; 2015. p. 150–7.
6. Bonnefoy-Mazure A, Armand S. Normal gait. In: Canavese F, Deslandes J, editors. Orthopedic management of children with cerebral palsy; 2015. p. 199–214.
7. McGraw B, McClenaghan BA, Williams HG, Dickerson J, Ward DS. Gait and postural stability in obese and nonobese prepubertal boys. Arch Phys Med Rehabil. 2000;81(4):484–9.
8. Lai PP, Leung AK, Li AN, Zhang M. Three-dimensional gait analysis of obese adults. Clin Biomech (Bristol, Avon). 2008;23(Suppl 1):S2–6.
9. Capodaglio P, Gobbi M, Donno L, Fumagalli A, Buratto C, Galli M, et al. Effect of obesity on knee and ankle biomechanics during walking. Sensors (Basel). 2021;21(21):7114.
10. Runhaar J, Koes BW, Clockaerts S, Bierma-Zeinstra SM. A systematic review on changed biomechanics of lower extremities in obese individuals: a possible role in development of osteoarthritis. Obes Rev. 2011;12(12):1071–82.
11. Walsh TP, Arnold JB, Evans AM, Yaxley A, Damarell RA, Shanahan EM. The association between body fat and musculoskeletal pain: a systematic review and meta-analysis. BMC Musculoskelet Disord. 2018;19(1):233.
12. Butterworth PA, Landorf KB, Smith SE, Menz HB. The association between body mass index and musculoskeletal foot disorders: a systematic review. Obes Rev. 2012;13(7):630–42.
13. Tanamas SK, Wluka AE, Berry P, Menz HB, Strauss BJ, Davies-Tuck M, et al. Relationship between obesity and foot pain and its association with fat mass, fat distribution, and muscle mass. Arthritis Care Res (Hoboken). 2012;64(2):262–8.
14. Dufour AB, Losina E, Menz HB, LaValley MP, Hannan MT. Obesity, foot pain and foot disorders in older men and women. Obes Res Clin Pract. 2017;11(4):445–53.
15. Butterworth PA, Urquhart DM, Landorf KB, Wluka AE, Cicuttini FM, Menz HB. Foot posture, range of motion and plantar pressure characteristics in obese and non-obese individuals. Gait Posture. 2015;41(2):465–9.
16. Angin S, Crofts G, Mickle KJ, Nester CJ. Ultrasound evaluation of foot muscles and plantar fascia in pes planus. Gait Posture. 2014;40(1):48–52.
17. Mickle KJ, Munro BJ, Lord SR, Menz HB, Steele JR. Foot pain, plantar pressures, and falls in older people: a prospective study. J Am Geriatr Soc. 2010;58(10):1936–40.
18. Wearing SC, Hennig EM, Byrne NM, Steele JR, Hills AP. Musculoskeletal disorders associated with obesity: a biomechanical perspective. Obes Rev. 2006;7(3):239–50.
19. Dina OA, Green PG, Levine JD. Role of interleukin-6 in chronic muscle hyperalgesic priming. Neuroscience. 2008;152(2):521–5.
20. Riddle DL, Pulisic M, Pidcoe P, Johnson RE. Risk factors for plantar fasciitis: a matched case-control study. J Bone Joint Surg Am. 2003;85(5):872–7.
21. van Leeuwen KD, Rogers J, Winzenberg T, van Middelkoop M. Higher body mass index is associated with plantar fasciopathy/'plantar fasciitis': systematic review and meta-analysis of various clinical and imaging risk factors. Br J Sports Med. 2016;50(16):972–81.
22. Taş S, Bek N, Ruhi Onur M, Korkusuz F. Effects of body mass index on mechanical properties of the plantar fascia and heel pad in asymptomatic participants. Foot Ankle Int. 2017;38(7):779–84.

23. Chen W-M, Lee PV-S. Explicit finite element modelling of heel pad mechanics in running: inclusion of body dynamics and application of physiological impact loads. Comput Methods Biomech Biomed Engin. 2015;18(14):1582–95.
24. Rome K, Campbell R, Flint A, Haslock I. Heel pad thickness—a contributing factor associated with plantar heel pain in young adults. Foot Ankle Int. 2002;23(2):142–7.
25. Cheung JT-M, Zhang M, An K-N. Effects of plantar fascia stiffness on the biomechanical responses of the ankle–foot complex. Clin Biomech. 2004;19(8):839–46.
26. Gaida JE, Ashe MC, Bass SL, Cook JL. Is adiposity an under-recognized risk factor for tendinopathy? A systematic review. Arthritis Rheum. 2009;61(6):840–9.
27. Weil L. Obesity, feet, and the impact on health care. Foot Ankle Spec. 2012;5(3):148–9.
28. Abate M. How obesity modifies tendons (implications for athletic activities). Muscles Ligaments Tendons J. 2014;4(3):298–302.
29. Battery L, Maffulli N. Inflammation in overuse tendon injuries. Sports Med Arthrosc Rev. 2011;19(3):213–7.
30. Stolzman S, Irby MB, Callahan AB, Skelton JA. Pes planus and paediatric obesity: a systematic review of the literature. Clin Obes. 2015;5(2):52–9.
31. Mickle KJ, Steele JR, Munro BJ. The feet of overweight and obese young children: are they flat or fat? Obesity (Silver Spring). 2006;14(11):1949–53.
32. Reb CW, Schick FA, Karanjia HN, Daniel JN. High prevalence of obesity and female gender among patients with concomitant tibialis posterior tendonitis and plantar fasciitis. Foot Ankle Spec. 2015;8(5):364–8.
33. Irving DB, Cook JL, Young MA, Menz HB. Obesity and pronated foot type may increase the risk of chronic plantar heel pain: a matched case-control study. BMC Musculoskelet Disord. 2007;8:41.
34. Gross CE, Lampley A, Green CL, DeOrio JK, Easley M, Adams S, et al. The effect of obesity on functional outcomes and complications in total ankle arthroplasty. Foot Ankle Int. 2016;37(2):137–41.
35. Sansosti LE, Van JC, Meyr AJ. Effect of obesity on total ankle arthroplasty: a systematic review of postoperative complications requiring surgical revision. J Foot Ankle Surg. 2018;57(2):353–6.
36. Werner BC, Burrus MT, Looney AM, Park JS, Perumal V, Cooper MT. Obesity is associated with increased complications after operative management of end-stage ankle arthritis. Foot Ankle Int. 2015;36(8):863–70.

Obesity and Paediatric Disorders 10

Orna Alexandra Glynn, Eisten Keogh, and Ciara Egan

10.1 Introduction

Paediatric or childhood obesity is a global epidemic of considerable concern, particularly in the field of orthopaedics. The World Health Organization (WHO) estimates that worldwide 38.2 million children under the age of 5 years and over 340 million children aged between 5 and 19 years of age are overweight or obese. The prevalence of obesity amongst children has rapidly increased in recent decades, where over 18% of children between the ages of 5–9 years today are considered overweight or obese compared with just 4% in 1975 [1].

The bone mass attained in childhood and adolescence is an important modifiable factor in the development of lifelong skeletal health. Approximately 40–60% of adult bone mass is accrued during adolescence, and at the age of 18, 90% of peak bone mass occurs [2].

O. A. Glynn (✉)
National Orthopaedic Hospital Cappagh, Dublin, Ireland

E. Keogh
School of Medicine, Royal College of Surgeons in Ireland, Dublin, Ireland
e-mail: eistenkeogh20@rcsi.com

C. Egan
Children's Health Ireland, Crumlin, Dublin, Ireland

J. M. O´Byrne et al. (eds.), *Musculoskeletal Disease and Obesity*,
https://doi.org/10.1007/978-3-031-63310-2_10

Skeletal deficiencies that occur in childhood and adolescence may persist throughout life. Therefore, intervention at this stage is critical in improving the future bone health of this generation. Obesity plays an important role in bone health as increased adiposity has a negative effect on achieving peak bone mass [3]. According to Wolff's law [4], healthy bone will adapt to the loads under which it is placed and loading to a particular bone will result in remodelling so that the bone may become stronger to resist those forces. Therefore, children with increased body mass and an associated increased stressing of the bones should result in increased bone density. Multiple studies have shown that obese children have greater bone strength, greater bone mineral density for height, larger bones, increased vertebral density, increased height, and earlier maturation [3]. Despite this, various nutritional deficiencies as well as endocrine-related changes associated with obesity lead to an overall decrease in relative bone mass, when the actual body weight is taken into account [5].

10.2 Obesity and Bone Metabolism

Mechanisms involving adipose tissue in bone metabolism are complex, not least because fat cells and osteoblasts are both derived from MSC in the bone marrow [6]. Osteoclasts originate from monocyte/macrophage precursors of the myeloid lineage of hematopoietic stem cells [6]. Once formed, adipocytes and macrophages secrete several cytokines such as tumour necrosis factor-α (TNF-α), interleukin-1β (IL-1β), and interleukin-6 (IL-6), which are capable of stimulating osteoclast activity and bone resorption via regulation of the RANKL/RANK/OPG pathway. OPG, a decoy receptor secreted by preosteoblasts, acts as a decoy receptor to RANKL, and therefore, inhibits osteoclast activation and bone resorption (Fig. 10.1).

Child and adolescent overweight/obesity are linked with vitamin D deficiency [7]. These negative effects are primarily attributed to the action of vitamin D on glycaemic control. The biological mechanisms involved are not well understood but are proposed to include enhancing glucose uptake through both direct and indirect means, regulation of glucose-mediated secretion of insulin by pancreatic beta cells, and reducing inflammation [8].

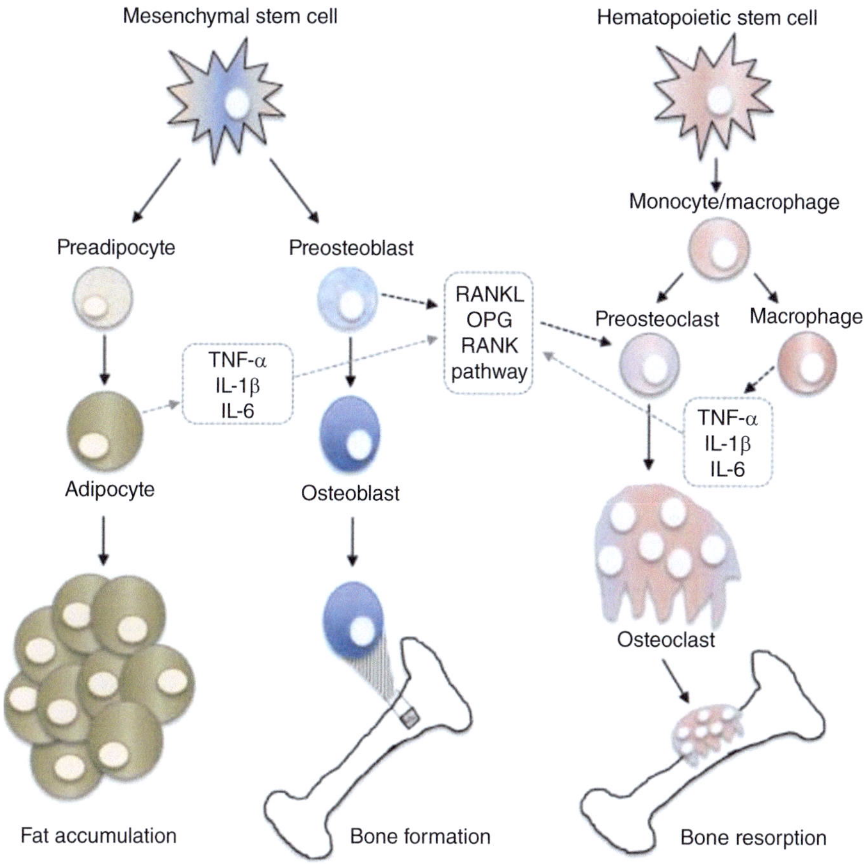

Fig. 10.1 Complex interactions between fat accumulation, bone formation, and bone resorption [6]. (Reproduced with permission from Elsevier)

10.3 Patterns of Injuries

Obesity is associated with an increased incidence of childhood fractures. A Spanish study of 450,000 children concluded that obese children at the time of starting school had a 70% and 20% increased risk of lower limb and upper limb fractures during childhood, respectively, while children with an overweight BMI had increased risks of 40% and 10% [9]. There is a significantly greater force generated by an overweight child compared to a healthy-weight child when they fall on an outstretched limb [10]. This leads to an increased risk of fracture from low-fall heights and when landing on softer-impact surfaces [10].

Overweight children also report poorer mobility [10], and balance [11], and as such may also be more likely to suffer awkward falls, compared to their active, nimble counterparts. The combination of these factors with the increased force generated by the increased body mass leads to increased risk of fracture, particularly with falls onto outstretched limbs [10].

Obese children often present with different and more complex fracture patterns. Pollack et al. found the rate of injury following motor accidents to be similar between overweight/obese and normal BMI children [12]. However, higher BMI children had a higher rate of distal extremity fractures [12]. They hypothesised that increased extremity mass combined with the increased proximity to internal vehicle structures led to increased velocity on impact. In another study, Pomerantz et al. concluded that, compared to normal BMI children, obese children are more likely to suffer lower extremity injuries than upper extremity injuries and are less likely to suffer face and head injuries than their normal-weight peers [13].

In a recent review of paediatric elbow fractures, a higher rate of obesity was detected in the lateral condyle fracture cohort compared with the supracondylar fracture cohort. Fornari et al. suggested that due to the known limitation in mobility and balance associated with higher weight and adiposity, these children struggled to sufficiently brace their falls on a fully extended arm [14]. In this situation, varus stress is applied to a partially flexed elbow, resulting in a lateral condyle fracture. Within the lateral condyle fracture cohort, those patients with higher BMI also demonstrated higher degrees of displacement and articular involvement. This higher degree of injury complexity and severity has also been demonstrated in supracondylar fractures, with those occurring in obese children resulting in higher rates of neurovascular complications and increased fracture pattern complexity [15]. Furthermore, Li et al. found that obese children were four times more likely to require open reduction of supracondylar fractures [16]. This increased requirement is likely due to a combination of difficulty in fracture manipulation caused by excess subcutaneous fat, as well as increased fracture complexity [15].

The rate of physical injuries in lower extremity fractures is more than twice as high in obese children as normal-weight children following blunt trauma. Gilbert et al. theorised that this is due to a combination of the physiological effects of obesity on the physis and the increased force generated with the injury due to increased body mass [17].

10.4 Challenges in Fracture Management in Obese Children

There are many challenges posed by obesity in the management of paediatric fractures. As previously discussed, overweight and obese children are more likely to suffer neurovascular complications and more complex fracture patterns [15]. The presence of increased adiposity interferes with traditional methods of managing paediatric fractures, namely, the application of a well-moulded cast. Where immobilisation was previously a suitable primary option for managing paediatric fractures, increasing rates of childhood obesity are now resulting in failed treatment with casting, requiring repeated manipulations or surgical fixation. The cornerstone of successful cast treatment depends on the cast ability to control the injured bone underlying. Increased adiposity leads to an overall increase in the size of the soft-tissue envelope, increasing the distance from the cast to the bone. This leads to difficulty in controlling fracture fragments and maintaining fracture reduction [3]. While achieving an optimum cast index in obese children is possible, it may be more difficult. In the management of paediatric both bone forearm fractures [18], overweight and obese children had a 16% increased risk of failing non-surgical management. Another study reported that overweight children were six times more likely to lose reduction compared to non-overweight children [19]. The rate of displacement requiring repeated manipulation or surgical fixation in distal radius fracture is also significantly higher in obese patients [20]. Due to this proven difficulty in maintaining fracture reduction in a cast, obese children presenting with unstable fractures should undergo closer surveillance if cast immobilisation is chosen as the method of treatment. Parents of these children should also be counselled on the increased risk of reduction loss, requiring possible surgical fixation. Consideration should also be given to proceeding directly to surgical fixation in the form of percutaneous pinning, on a case-by-case basis.

10.4.1 Anaesthetic Risks

The use of sedation and anaesthetic agents in obese children can result in higher rates of complications compared to use in normal-weight patients. This is due to the volume of distribution, most notably in inhaled agents, being altered. Many drugs used commonly in sedation are lipid soluble. Therefore, in the presence of increased amounts of adipose tissue, the metabolism of these drugs can be unpredictable [21]. Dosing can also be challenging in this cohort as recommended doses are based on ideal body weight as opposed to total body weight [21]. When examining patients with long bone fractures requiring sedation for reduction, Hirsch et al. found that obese patients suffered twice the oxygen desaturation rates as non-obese patients [22]. Obesity is associated with an overall reduction in respiratory function, as well as increased rates of sleep apnoea and asthma. Sleep apnoea, in particular, can lead to difficulty during intubation and affects 2% of all children. Anaesthesiologists or other healthcare providers managing these cases need to appreciate the physiological differences in obese children as they often require prolonged ventilation due to acute respiratory failure [23]. Comorbidities such as hypertension, type II diabetes mellitus, and bronchial asthma are more common in overweight and obese children. Surgeons should consider optimising these conditions preoperatively, particularly in the setting of elective procedures [24].

10.4.2 Perioperative Risks

Many studies have been carried out in the assessment of perioperative complications in obese paediatric patients. Children with abnormal body weight, either overweight or underweight, are at a higher risk of developing surgical-site infections [25].

Georgopoulos et al. studied the risk of venous thromboembolism (VTE) in paediatric orthopaedic patients following elective surgery, and while the overall incidence of deep vein thrombosis (DVT) and pulmonary embolism (PE) was low (5.1 per 10,000 admissions), factors such as increasing age, those who had other complications associated with a surgical procedure or an implanted device, and any obese patients or patients with metabolic syndrome were at an increased risk of developing VTE (6.1 times the rate in the general population). Of this accumulated group of patients, 25% were obese [26]. When assessing the risk factors for injuries following trauma in obese paediatric patients, Rana et al. concluded that these patients were at a higher risk of developing deep vein thrombosis, as well as decubitus ulcers, than normal-weight children [27].

In patients 18 years and younger undergoing peri-acetabular osteotomy, Nouvais et al. concluded that obese patients have a ten-fold increased risk of developing postoperative complications. The most common complications included superficial and deep infections, and wound haematomas [28]. Obese patients who underwent fixation for femur fractures also developed higher rates of complications, including wound infection, osteomyelitis, malunion, wound dehiscence, broken implants, and compartment syndrome [29, 30].

Upasani et al. evaluated postoperative morbidity in obese and non-obese adolescents who underwent surgery for scoliosis. Obese patients had longer operative times, increased intraoperative blood loss, and increased intraoperative intravenous fluid requirements [31].

An evaluation of patients who required a return to the operating theatre within 90 days of initial spinal fusion found that the only factor related to an increased risk of infection was BMI percent for age. This was attributed to the underlying impairment in systemic function caused by obesity, including hemastatic function, metabolic changes, and cardiorespiratory dysfunction [32].

10.4.3 Implant-Related Complications

Implant failure is a complication that occurs at higher rates when treating obese paediatric patients. This has been demonstrated most notably in guided growth techniques. In a member survey carried out by Burghardt et al. with the Paediatric Orthopaedic Society of North America, 15% of the members reported implant failure. Of these failures, 93% of the patients were overweight or obese [33]. Failures were attributed to the cannulated nature of the screws. As a result, many surgeons have turned to the use of solid screws in conjunction with plates with options for multiple screws on either side of the physis in the treatment of angular deformities [3] in the obese population.

10.5 Obesity-Related Paediatric Orthopaedic Conditions

10.5.1 Blount's Disease

Blount's disease is an acquired asymmetrical growth disorder of the medial proximal tibia that results in a three-dimensional deformity that includes genu varum, procurvatum, and internal tibial rotation [34, 35]. There are two clinical variants of this disease, depending on when signs develop. The exact aetiology of Blount's disease is unknown. However, development of disease is likely to be multifactorial, consisting of genetic predisposition, increased mechanical pressure on the growth plate due to obesity and/or early ambulation, as well as nutritional status [35]. Early-onset Blount's disease typically arises in children between 1 and 3 years of age, typically in those who have ambulated early (before 10 months of age) [34]. If left untreated, irreversible asymmetric epiphysiodesis develop on the medial proximal tibia around 6–8 years of age, and knee deformities deteriorate gradually. Spontaneous resolution can occur, but this is less likely in overweight or obese children. In most cases, conservative or operative intervention is required. Conservative treatment involves the use of braces that apply valgus force to the knee and are an option for children under the age of 3 years. However, they are not used routinely due to the difficultly with compliance. Surgical intervention depends on the patient age and disease severity. Early guided growth can be of use; however, deformity correction with mechanical axis realignment is often required. Surgical intervention for advanced disease must be tailored to each individual case. Late-onset Blount's disease, occurring after the age of 10 years, predominantly affects obese or morbidly obese children. This presents a significant challenge for treatment, which aims to correct deformities, improve function, and decrease the risk of premature osteoarthritis. Options include a lateral hemi-epiphysiodesis or corrective osteotomy [34].

10.5.2 Slipped Capital Femoral Epiphysis

Slipped capital femoral epiphysis typically affects adolescents who present complaining of atraumatic knee, thigh, or hip pain which may be associated with a limp [36]. The classic clinical finding is of obligate external rotation in flexion. The change in the relationship of the femoral head and shaft due to the slip causes a complex 3D deformity. The incidence of SCFE is increasing worldwide, concurrent with the global childhood obesity epidemic [37]. Obesity is a major risk factor for SCFE development, with a temporal, dose–response relationship demonstrated in the literature. For instance, severe obesity in children aged 11–12 years is associated with a 17 times greater risk than those children with a normal BMI. Furthermore, bilateral SCFE is occurring more frequently than previously. A reduction in BMI has been shown to lower the risk of the development of bilateral SCFE [38].

SCFE causes significant disability in childhood, but is also potentially associated with profound lifelong disability due to the abnormal femoral head shape, including hip joint impingement and premature osteoarthritis. Due to their obesity, these children are also at a higher lifetime risk of hypothyroidism and have a higher risk of all-cause mortality compared with individuals without SCFE [39]. Initial operative treatment for SCFE is required to prevent progression of the slip. Single-screw fixation of the lesser grades of slip is the most widely accepted treatment due to its high success rate, limited soft-tissue injury, and low incidence of complications of osteonecrosis or chondrolysis [36]. Secondary procedures are often required to reorient the femoral head once the initial injury has healed. The correct management of high-grade acute slips remains an area of debate.

10.5.3 Legg–Calvé–Perthes Disease (LCPD)

LCPD is an idiopathic avascular necrosis of the epiphysis of the femoral head, typically affecting children between 5 and 7 years of age. It occurs predominantly in boys, with a male-to-female ratio of 5:1 [40, 41]. No consensus has been reached about its exact aetiology; however, recent evidence supports obesity and increased leptin levels as the major risk factors [42, 43], and both are positively associated with disease severity. It is postulated that increased levels of circulating leptin in obese children lead to bone remodelling, resulting in ischaemic necrosis of the femoral head. Moreover, it suggests that leptin resistance in LCPD reduces revascularisation and is associated with poor treatment outcomes [43]. This recent research diverts from the 'classic' view of an LCPD patient, who was described as being thin, small, and socio-economically disadvantaged [44]. The aetiology of LCDP may also be explained by interference with normal blood supply to the epiphysis due to repetitive mechanical stress [44, 45]. Hypertension may also be an aetiological factor [46], as the prevalence of hypertension was found to be higher in children with LCPD compared with the general paediatric population. Treatment for LCPD depends on the patient age and stage of disease at presentation [47].

10.6 Interventions

10.6.1 Preoperative Optimisation

Childhood obesity is associated with several medical comorbidities. The most significant of these include bronchial asthma, sleep apnoea, hypertension, hypercholesterolemia, and type II diabetes mellitus [48]. Depending on the severity or control of the condition, these processes can lead to significant peri- and postoperative morbidity, ranging from anaesthetic- and airway-related complications, to postoperative surgical-site infections. Prior to elective procedures, specialist referral to pulmonary and endocrine physicians should be considered in order to optimise medical comorbidities. 'At-risk' patients identified should also be seen at a pre-assessment clinic with review by an anaesthesiologist prior to undergoing elective procedures [24].

Vitamin D screening is advised prior to major elective procedures in obese children, who are typically deficient in this mineral [49]. Sufficient vitamin D levels are required for full recovery following orthopaedic procedures, particularly in those involving guided growth techniques, osteotomies, or posterior spinal fusion for scoliosis [49].

Obese children are significantly more likely to develop venous thromboembolic complications following orthopaedic procedures [26]. For this reason, all members of this cohort should be assessed with regards to VTE risk on admission to hospital, with particular attention paid to post-pubertal adolescents. Appropriate VTE prophylaxis should be determined according to patient-specific risk factors, as outlined by the Association of Paediatric Anaesthetists of Great Britain & Ireland.

The Orthopaedic Clinic may be the first point of contact in the hospital setting for some of these children. Orthopaedic surgeons have a duty to their patients and the wider healthcare team to address obesity amongst the paediatric population, particularly when its effect on MSK health is considered. This may be in the form of simple lifestyle advice when the opportunity arises in clinics. This should include, but should not be limited to, dietary advice, liaising with primary care physicians to arrange appropriate follow-up, dietician referral, promotion of active lifestyle, and counselling of patients and parents on the orthopaedic risks associated with obesity.

10.7 Conclusions

- Childhood obesity affects bone quality in a manner which may have lifelong consequences.
- This is due in part to the metabolic effect on the growing bone but also to the orthopaedic conditions associated with obesity.
- These children are more likely to have more complex fracture patterns and a higher rate of primary and perioperative complications.
- Deformity caused by conditions such as SCFE and Blount's which are more common in obese children can lead to early joint degeneration.
- An awareness of the perioperative complications in this group allows preventative measures to be put in place and also informs the consent process.
- Understanding the potential long-term medical problems which this cohort faces makes it more likely that early onward referral to active management of obesity will occur.
- Quick interventions with advice on vitamin D intake and encouragement of an active lifestyle should be considered at the orthopaedic outpatient clinic.

References

1. WHO. Obesity and overweight 2021 Available from: https://www.who.int/news-room/fact-sheets/detail/obesity-and-overweight.
2. Golden NH, Abrams SA, Committee on Nutrition, Daniels SR, Abrams SA, Corkins MR, et al. Optimizing bone health in children and adolescents. Pediatrics. 2014;134(4):e1229–43. https://doi.org/10.1542/peds.2014-2173.
3. Nowicki P, Kemppainen J, Maskill L, Cassidy J. The role of obesity in pediatric orthopedics. J Am Acad Orthop Surg Glob Res Rev. 2019;3(5):e036. https://doi.org/10.5435/JAAOSGlobal-D-19-00036.
4. Wolff J. The law of bone remodeling. Berlin: Springer-Verlag; 1986. https://doi.org/10.1007/978-3-642-71031-5. [1892].
5. Bialo SR, Gordon CM. Underweight, overweight, and pediatric bone fragility: impact and management. Curr Osteoporos Rep. 2014;12(3):319–28. https://doi.org/10.1007/s11914-014-0226-z.
6. Pollock NK. Childhood obesity, bone development, and cardiometabolic risk factors. Mol Cell Endocrinol. 2015;410:52–63. https://doi.org/10.1016/j.mce.2015.03.016.
7. Fiamenghi VI, Mello ED. Vitamin D deficiency in children and adolescents with obesity: a meta-analysis. J Pediatr. 2021;97(3):273–9. https://doi.org/10.1016/j.jped.2020.08.006.
8. Stivelman E, Retnakaran R. Role of vitamin D in the pathophysiology and treatment of type 2 diabetes. Curr Diabetes Rev. 2012;8(1):42–7. https://doi.org/10.2174/157339912798829179.
9. Lane JC, Butler KL, Poveda-Marina JL, Martinez-Laguna D, Reyes C, de Bont J, et al. Preschool obesity is associated with an increased risk of childhood fracture: a longitudinal cohort study of 466,997 children and up to 11 years of follow-up in Catalonia, Spain. J Bone Miner Res. 2020;35(6):1022–30. https://doi.org/10.1002/jbmr.3984.
10. Taylor ED, Theim KR, Mirch MC, Ghorbani S, Tanofsky-Kraff M, Adler-Wailes DC, et al. Orthopedic complications of overweight in children and adolescents. Pediatrics. 2006;117(6):2167–74. https://doi.org/10.1542/peds.2005-1832.
11. Goulding A, Jones IE, Taylor RW, Piggot JM, Taylor D. Dynamic and static tests of balance and postural sway in boys: effects of previous wrist bone fractures and high adiposity. Gait Posture. 2003;17(2):136–41. https://doi.org/10.1016/s0966-6362(02)00161-3.
12. Pollack KM, Xie D, Arbogast KB, Durbin DR. Body mass index and injury risk among US children 9-15 years old in motor vehicle crashes. Inj Prev. 2008;14(6):366–71. https://doi.org/10.1136/ip.2008.019208.
13. Pomerantz WJ, Timm NL, Gittelman MA. Injury patterns in obese versus nonobese children presenting to a pediatric emergency department. Pediatrics. 2010;125(4):681–5. https://doi.org/10.1542/peds.2009-2367.
14. Fornari ED, Suszter M, Roocroft J, Bastrom T, Edmonds EW, Schlechter J. Childhood obesity as a risk factor for lateral condyle fractures over supracondylar humerus fractures. Clin Orthop Relat Res. 2013;471(4):1193–8. https://doi.org/10.1007/s11999-012-2566-2.
15. Seeley MA, Gagnier JJ, Srinivasan RC, Hensinger RN, VanderHave KL, Farley FA, et al. Obesity and its effects on pediatric supracondylar humeral fractures. J Bone Joint Surg Am. 2014;96(3):e18. https://doi.org/10.2106/jbjs.L.01643.
16. Li NY, Bruce WJ, Joyce C, Decker NM, Cappello T. Obesity's influence on operative management of pediatric supracondylar humerus fractures. J Pediatr Orthop. 2018;38(3):e118–21. https://doi.org/10.1097/bpo.0000000000001126.
17. Gilbert SR, MacLennan PA, Backstrom I, Creek A, Sawyer J. Altered lower extremity fracture characteristics in obese pediatric trauma patients. J Orthop Trauma. 2015;29(1):e12–7. https://doi.org/10.1097/bot.0000000000000132.
18. Okoroafor UC, Cannada LK, McGinty JL. Obesity and failure of nonsurgical management of pediatric both-bone forearm fractures. J Hand Surg Am. 2017;42(9):711–6. https://doi.org/10.1016/j.jhsa.2017.06.006.

19. DeFrancesco CJ, Rogers BH, Shah AS. Obesity increases risk of loss of reduction after casting for diaphyseal fractures of the radius and ulna in children: an observational cohort study. J Orthop Trauma. 2018;32(2):e46–51. https://doi.org/10.1097/bot.0000000000001010.
20. Auer RT, Mazzone P, Robinson L, Nyland J, Chan G. Childhood obesity increases the risk of failure in the treatment of distal forearm fractures. J Pediatr Orthop. 2016;36(8):e86–e8. https://doi.org/10.1097/bpo.0000000000000649.
21. Samuels PJ, Sjoblom MD. Anesthetic considerations for pediatric obesity and adolescent bariatric surgery. Curr Opin Anaesthesiol. 2016;29(3):327–36. https://doi.org/10.1097/aco.0000000000000330.
22. Hirsch DG, Tyo J, Wrotniak BH. Desaturation in procedural sedation for children with long bone fractures: does weight status matter? Am J Emerg Med. 2017;35(8):1060–3. https://doi.org/10.1016/j.ajem.2017.02.036.
23. Lazar-Antman MA, Leet AI. Effects of obesity on pediatric fracture care and management. J Bone Joint Surg Am. 2012;94(9):855–61. https://doi.org/10.2106/jbjs.J.01839.
24. Nafiu OO, Reynolds PI, Bamgbade OA, Tremper KK, Welch K, Kasa-Vubu JZ. Childhood body mass index and perioperative complications. Paediatr Anaesth. 2007;17(5):426–30. https://doi.org/10.1111/j.1460-9592.2006.02140.x.
25. Blackwood BP, Gause CD, Harris JC, Theodorou CM, Helenowski I, Lautz TB, et al. Overweight and obese pediatric patients have an increased risk of developing a surgical site infection. Surg Infect. 2017;18(4):491–7. https://doi.org/10.1089/sur.2016.179.
26. Georgopoulos G, Hotchkiss MS, McNair B, Siparsky G, Carry PM, Miller NH. Incidence of deep vein thrombosis and pulmonary embolism in the elective pediatric orthopaedic patient. J Pediatr Orthop. 2016;36(1):101–9. https://doi.org/10.1097/bpo.0000000000000391.
27. Rana AR, Michalsky MP, Teich S, Groner JI, Caniano DA, Schuster DP. Childhood obesity: a risk factor for injuries observed at a level-1 trauma center. J Pediatr Surg. 2009;44(8):1601–5. https://doi.org/10.1016/j.jpedsurg.2008.11.060.
28. Novais EN, Potter GD, Sierra RJ, Kim YJ, Clohisy JC, Schoenecker PL, et al. Surgical treatment of adolescent acetabular dysplasia with a periacetabular osteotomy: does obesity increase the risk of complications? J Pediatr Orthop. 2015;35(6):561–4. https://doi.org/10.1097/bpo.0000000000000327.
29. Leet AI, Pichard CP, Ain MC. Surgical treatment of femoral fractures in obese children: does excessive body weight increase the rate of complications? J Bone Joint Surg Am. 2005;87(12):2609–13. https://doi.org/10.2106/jbjs.D.02019.
30. Weiss JM, Choi P, Ghatan C, Skaggs DL, Kay RM. Complications with flexible nailing of femur fractures more than double with child obesity and weight >50 kg. J Child Orthop. 2009;3(1):53–8. https://doi.org/10.1007/s11832-008-0149-2.
31. Upasani VV, Caltoum C, Petcharaporn M, Bastrom T, Pawelek J, Marks M, et al. Does obesity affect surgical outcomes in adolescent idiopathic scoliosis? Spine (Phila Pa 1976). 2008;33(3):295–300. https://doi.org/10.1097/BRS.0b013e3181624573.
32. Newton PO, Bastrom TP, Yaszay B. Patient-specific risk adjustment improves comparison of infection rates following posterior fusion for adolescent idiopathic scoliosis. J Bone Joint Surg Am. 2017;99(21):1846–50. https://doi.org/10.2106/jbjs.16.01442.
33. Burghardt RD, Specht SC, Herzenberg JE. Mechanical failures of eight-plateguided growth system for temporary hemiepiphysiodesis. J Pediatr Orthop. 2010;30(6):594–7. https://doi.org/10.1097/BPO.0b013e3181e4f591.
34. Janoyer M. Blount disease. Orthop Traumatol Surg Res. 2019;105(1s):S111–21. https://doi.org/10.1016/j.otsr.2018.01.009.
35. Banwarie RR, Hollman F, Meijs N, Arts JJ, Vroemen P, Moh P, et al. Insight into the possible aetiologies of Blount's disease: a systematic review of the literature. J Pediatr Orthop B. 2020;29(4):323–36. https://doi.org/10.1097/bpb.0000000000000677.
36. Aronsson DD, Loder RT, Breur GJ, Weinstein SL. Slipped capital femoral epiphysis: current concepts. J Am Acad Orthop Surg. 2006;14(12):666–79. https://doi.org/10.5435/00124635-200611000-00010.

37. Perry DC, Metcalfe D, Lane S, Turner S. Childhood obesity and slipped capital femoral epiphysis. Pediatrics. 2018;142(5):e20181067. https://doi.org/10.1542/peds.2018-1067.
38. Nasreddine AY, Heyworth BE, Zurakowski D, Kocher MS. A reduction in body mass index lowers risk for bilateral slipped capital femoral epiphysis. Clin Orthop Relat Res. 2013;471(7):2137–44. https://doi.org/10.1007/s11999-013-2811-3.
39. Hailer YD. Fate of patients with slipped capital femoral epiphysis (SCFE) in later life: risk of obesity, hypothyroidism, and death in 2,564 patients with SCFE compared with 25,638 controls. Acta Orthop. 2020;91(4):457–63. https://doi.org/10.1080/17453674.2020.1749810.
40. Loder RT, Skopelja EN. The epidemiology and demographics of legg-calvé-perthes' disease. ISRN Orthop. 2011;2011:504393. https://doi.org/10.5402/2011/504393.
41. Perry DC, Hall AJ. The epidemiology and etiology of Perthes disease. Orthop Clin North Am. 2011;42(3):279–83. https://doi.org/10.1016/j.ocl.2011.03.002.
42. Neal DC, Alford TH, Moualeu A, Jo CH, Herring JA, Kim HK. Prevalence of obesity in patients with Legg-Calvé-Perthes disease. J Am Acad Orthop Surg. 2016;24(9):660–5. https://doi.org/10.5435/jaaos-d-16-00120.
43. Lee JH, Zhou L, Kwon KS, Lee D, Park BH, Kim JR. Role of leptin in Legg-Calvé-Perthes disease. J Orthop Res. 2013;31(10):1605–10. https://doi.org/10.1002/jor.22415.
44. Pavone V, Chisari E, Vescio A, Lizzio C, Sessa G, Testa G. Aetiology of Legg-Calvé-Perthes disease: a systematic review. World J Orthop. 2019;10(3):145–65. https://doi.org/10.5312/wjo.v10.i3.145.
45. Guerado E, Caso E. The physiopathology of avascular necrosis of the femoral head: an update. Injury. 2016;47(Suppl 6):S16–26. https://doi.org/10.1016/s0020-1383(16)30835-x.
46. Mörlin GB, Hailer YD. High blood pressure and overweight in children with Legg-Calvé-Perthes disease: a nationwide population-based cohort study. BMC Musculoskelet Disord. 2021;22(1):32. https://doi.org/10.1186/s12891-020-03889-9.
47. Maleki A, Qoreishy SM, Bahrami MN. Surgical treatments for Legg-Calvé-Perthes disease: comprehensive review. Interact J Med Res. 2021;10(2):e27075. https://doi.org/10.2196/27075.
48. Pulgarón ER. Childhood obesity: a review of increased risk for physical and psychological comorbidities. Clin Ther. 2013;35(1):A18–32. https://doi.org/10.1016/j.clinthera.2012.12.014.
49. Clarke NM, Page JE. Vitamin D deficiency: a paediatric orthopaedic perspective. Curr Opin Pediatr. 2012;24(1):46–9. https://doi.org/10.1097/MOP.0b013e32834ec8eb.

11 Obesity and Musculoskeletal Oncology

Orna Alexandra Glynn, Allison Kelliher, Gary C. O'Toole, and Alan P. Molloy

11.1 Introduction

The International Agency for Research on Cancer (IARC) working group has stated that increased rates of adiposity are associated with increased incidences of certain cancers (in particular hormonally influenced cancers such as breast, ovarian and endometrial).

Various theories have been postulated for this link. One in particular describes the evidence that increased adipose tissue is associated with increased levels of oestrogen. This, in turn, is associated with increased risk of developing breast, ovarian and endometrial cancers.

Recent cancer statistics in the United States have claimed that 4.7% and 9.6% of male and female cancers, respectively, can be attributed to higher levels of body fat. Although there is no direct causal link between appendicular sarcomas and obesity, it is felt that uterine sarcomas are found in an increased incidence in those with an increased body mass index (BMI).

The main concerns with obesity in orthopaedic oncology are surgical exposure, delays in diagnoses and postoperative complications.

11.2 Surgical Exposure

Obtaining negative margins is paramount in orthopaedic oncology. The tumour should, taking anatomic constraints into account, be surrounded by a normal cuff of tissue. Achieving this is made easier with adequate surgical exposure.

O. A. Glynn · A. Kelliher · G. C. O'Toole · A. P. Molloy (✉)
National Orthopaedic Hospital Cappagh, Dublin, Ireland
e-mail: ornaalexandraglynn@rcsi.ie; allisonkelliher@rcsi.ie

J. M. O´Byrne et al. (eds.), *Musculoskeletal Disease and Obesity*,
https://doi.org/10.1007/978-3-031-63310-2_11

From positioning the patient to surgical incision and dissection, the goals of orthopaedic oncology can be made more difficult in the obese patient.

Positioning a patient in any surgery is vital for subsequent surgical exposure. In the obese patient with an abdominal apron, normal positioning for a groin dissection or pelvic surgery may have to be altered to adjust for body habitus. This, in turn, may necessitate an alteration in the surgical routine.

Incisions in orthopaedic oncology should be at least twice if not three times the length of the tumour. In patients with increased body fat, this may need to be lengthened accordingly. In the setting of neoadjuvant chemotherapy or radiotherapy, larger wounds can be associated with wound complications. We do not hesitate in making large incisions in orthopaedic oncology, but if certain factors are modifiable (increased BMI), this should be addressed.

Sarcomas, both soft tissue and primary bone, are often intimately associated with the adjacent neurovascular bundle. The en bloc resection of the tumour may necessitate the prior identification, protection and/or transposition of the vessels or nerves. This is technically easier in the thinner patient. With an increased soft-tissue envelope, there is anecdotal evidence of increased rates of iatrogenic injury to the adjacent structures.

11.3 Delays in Diagnoses

Obesity has been linked with an increased risk of multiple malignancies [1]. Furthermore, in patients with soft-tissue masses, it has also been suggested that obesity can contribute to a delay in diagnosis, with a potential effect on prognosis [2].

In breast cancer, obesity has been linked to increased tumour size, higher rates of lymphatic invasion and worse survival rates compared to normal-weight patients [3]. Similar to breast cancer, patients with soft-tissue sarcomas also often present with painless soft-tissue masses. In these patients, it has been suggested that the soft-tissue mass may be masked by the body habitus, thus presenting a potential barrier to early identification [2].

A further potential barrier to early diagnosis is the stigma associated with obesity, leading to embarrassment, low self-esteem and fear. This, as well as the association between lower socio-economic status and increased rates of obesity, can lead to delayed presentation to healthcare and poorer compliance with treatment [3].

In a study of 139 patients with soft-tissue sarcomas, Montgomery et al. found that obesity was associated with significantly larger tumour size at diagnosis in obese patients. They failed to identify an association between advanced tumour stage or worse survival rates in obese patients with soft-tissue sarcomas compared to the non-obese population [2].

However, the relationship between increased tumour size with both advanced stage and poorer prognosis has previously been demonstrated in a prospective analysis of 1,460 patients with both bone and soft-tissue sarcomas, with an 8.5-fold increased risk of death in patients found to have tumours measuring >25 cm compared to those with tumours <5 cm [4].

11.4 Complications

Obesity is associated with an increased incidence of surgical complications [5–7], and this finding is also reproducible in patients undergoing resections for soft-tissue sarcomas.

In his study, Montgomery et al. demonstrated a 3.5-fold increase in complication rate in obese patients compared to non-obese patients with similar tumour types and undergoing similar surgical procedures.

Excluding haematoma risk, obese patients were found to have higher rates of all other complications compared to patients with a body mass index of <30. This included infection (22% vs. 14%) and delayed healing (43% vs. 29%) [2].

Obese patients were also more likely to require complex wound closure techniques following resection of soft-tissue sarcomas, with 43% of obese patients requiring skin grafts, rotational or free flaps, or both, compared to just 25% in the non-obese cohort. This was attributed to increased tumour size, delays in wound healing, as well as the constellation of other complications observed more frequently in obese patients [2].

A study by Houdek et al. evaluated postoperative complications following lower extremity soft-tissue sarcoma resections in morbidly obese patients. They concluded that the presence of morbid obesity was related to significant increases in the rate of wound complications, infections and the requirement for repeated procedures (due to either wound complications or infection).

Other important factors included the use of preoperative radiation therapy, age >55 years, operative time >5 h and operations involving the foot or ankle. Of note, there was no significant difference in outcomes in terms of clear resection margins or recurrence (local or metastatic) between non-obese, obese and morbidly obese patients [8].

When evaluating patients who underwent upper extremity limb salvage surgery for soft-tissue sarcomas, Houdek et al. again found that morbidly obese patients (class III) were significantly higher rates of postoperative infections and wound-healing issues (dehiscence or delayed healing). This patient cohort was also strongly associated with a need for a repeated surgical procedure; however, this failed to reach statistical significance [9].

Montgomery et al. also evaluated rates of concurrent diabetes, tobacco use and use of an anticoagulant and found that obese patients had a significantly higher chance of having at least one of these comorbidities, of which diabetes was the most common. Current tobacco usage, as well as tumour location (groin, thigh or lower extremity), was associated with increased complications in both obese and non-obese patients [2].

11.5 Conclusion

Obesity has been noted to increase the risk of uterine sarcomas, although such a link has not been proven in the appendicular system. However, the risks of obesity in orthopaedic oncology are wide ranging and can be significant in certain cases.

These cases are time sensitive and therefore do not permit the use of many interventions preoperatively to address the issue. The risks associated with surgery for sarcomas in the obese patient should be noted and explained to the patient prior to surgery. The surgery is necessary and for the most part cannot be avoided (given the nature of the disease), but the patient must be aware of all the risks associated with their condition.

References

1. Wolk A, Gridley G, Svensson M, Nyren O, McLaughlin J, Fraumeni J, et al. A prospective study of obesity and cancer risk (Sweden). Cancer Causes Controls. 2001;12(1):13–21.
2. Montgomery C, Harris J, Siegel E, Suva L, Wilson M, Morell S, et al. Obesity is associated with larger soft-tissue sarcomas, more surgical complications, and more complex wound closures (obesity leads to larger soft-tissue sarcomas). J Surg Oncol. 2018;118(1):184–91.
3. Kyuwan L, Kruper L, Dieli-Conwright C, Mortimer J. The impact of obesity on breast cancer diagnosis and treatment. Curr Oncol Rep. 2019;21(5):41.
4. Grimer R. Size matters for sarcomas! Ann R Coll Surg Eng. 2006;88(6):519–24.
5. Hijazi H, Magne N, Levy A, Marcy P, Lacout A, Leysalle A, et al. Features of cancer management in obese patients. Crit Rev Oncol Hematol. 2013;85(2):193–205.
6. Hingorani P, Seidel K, Krailo M, Mascarenhas L, Meyers P, Marina N, et al. Body Mass Index (BMI) at diagnosis is associated with surgical wound complications in patients with localized osteosarcoma: a report from the Children's Oncology Group. Pediatr Blood Cancer. 2011;57(6):939–42.
7. McElroy M, Pivec R, Issa K, Harwin S, Mont M. The effects of obesity and morbid obesity on outcomes in TKA. J Knee Surg. 2013;26(2):83–8.
8. Houdek M, Hevesi M, Griffin A, Wunder J, Ferguson P. Morbid obesity is associated with an increased risk of wound complications and infection after lower extremity soft-tissue sarcoma resection. J Am Acad Orthop Surg. 2019;27(21):807–15.
9. Houdek M, Griffin A, Ferguson P, Wunder J. Morbid obesity increases the risk of postoperative wound complications, infection, and repeat surgical procedures following upper extremity limb salvage surgery for soft tissue sarcoma. AAHS. 2019;14(1):114–20.

Obesity and Sports Injuries

12

Ryan Alexander, Rosanne-Sara Lynham, and Brian M. Devitt

12.1 Introduction

The common colloquial term 'athletic physique' is often used to describe a fit, healthy and sporty individual. If we were to picture such an individual in our mind's eye, an image of a tall, slim, sinewed and muscled individual is likely to emerge. But as we know, athletes come in all shapes and sizes. What is more, modern athletes in their dedicated pursuit of the Olympic motto, faster-higher-stronger, have become quicker, taller and bigger. The advent of sports science has seen a paradigm shift in training methods for athletes, with world records being surpassed almost on an annual basis. The body shapes and composition of our athletes no longer reflect that of the general population and certainly pay little resemblance to the athletic population of the last two decades never mind the last century. Therefore, how relevant are the existing definitions we use to define body composition, especially obesity?

12.2 Defining Body Mass

In the context of scientific literature, the vast majority of authors use a standard body mass index (BMI) to measure participants' body composition [2–16]. The scale was originally created by Keys in 1972 to identify whether a person was underweight or overweight using the Quetelet Index [17]. The World Health Organization later classified the four quartiles of underweight (<18.5), normal (18.5–24.9), overweight (25–29.9) and obese (>30) [18]. However, a major limitation of this scale, which has been well documented, is its inability to

R. Alexander · R.-S. Lynham · B. M. Devitt (✉)
Dublin City University, UPMC Sports Surgery Clinic, Dublin, Ireland
e-mail: lynhamrs@tcd.ie; brian.devitt@dcu.ie

J. M. O´Byrne et al. (eds.), *Musculoskeletal Disease and Obesity*, https://doi.org/10.1007/978-3-031-63310-2_12

distinguish between body fat mass and body lean mass. Obesity, as a metabolic and anatomical measure, should indicate excess body fat yet those with a higher body lean mass will likely fall into the overweight or obese categories. Smalley et al. looked at this flaw in detail and found that men with a BMI of 27 (considered overweight) had body fat percentages of between 10% and 32% [19]. This body fat range included men with very lean physiques and those with an obese body fat percentage. This highlights the disparity between BMI and true body composition.

Notwithstanding this, the BMI scale appears to be used across various sporting populations, from elite athletes to adolescents. Some studies have used exact body mass and body types as a body composition measure when investigating a relationship with injury incidence [17, 18]. Kaplan et al. used an exact body mass figure in their study looking at the effect of body composition on injury risk in high school football players [17]. Whereas, Lee et al. classified participants via somatotyping, as well as BMI, in their study of rugby players [18]. Consequently, although BMI is the most popular method of body composition measurement and obesity is almost exclusively measured via BMI, we must consider these other methods of measurement when exploring the evidence with regards to injury.

In certain sports, a higher body mass is desirable. Examples of this include powerlifters, rugby players and American footballers. Fennell showed in a cohort study in under-20 rugby that 61/94 forwards across the 2022 Six Nations Championship had a BMI >30 [22]. Interestingly, none of the backs had a BMI >30, although with a mean BMI of 26.4, they would be considered in the 'overweight' category. In the NFL in 2005, 97% of players had a BMI >25, 56% had a BMI >30 and 26% had a BMI >35 [23]. In comparison to other sports, tennis players Rafael Nadal and Roger Federer had a BMI of 24.8, Liverpool FC had a team average BMI of 23.1 and the Kerry Gaelic Football team had an average BMI of 24.7 in 2022 [22]. Hence, we can see the variance in BMI depending on the sport.

If one were to consider the BMI levels of the rugby and NFL players in isolation, one might conclude that these players are, in fact, obese, and be at greater risk of medical complications associated with obesity [1]. However, fat-free mass and aerobic fitness are not taken into account within these figures. A 2018 study in youth male rugby players by Gavarry et al. investigated this blatant disparity. They stated that only 53% of players deemed overweight or obese by BMI had excess body fat using the body fat mass index (BFMI) [24]. Almost half of those deemed overweight or obese by BMI did not, in fact, have excess body fat. In young male handball players, BMI is typically high (25.1 ± 2.9) but their body fat percentage is within normal levels ($13.6 \pm 2.8\%$), indicating that fat-free mass is high in these players rather than body fat [25]. Fitness levels are also important to note as cardiovascular fitness has a large association with all-cause morbidity. Elite rugby union forwards were shown to have an average VO2Max of 48.3 ± 3.5 ml/kg/min, despite their 'obesity', whereas an inactive male will record a VO2Max of 35–40 ml/kg/min [26, 27]. Therefore, we can clearly see the difficulty in standardising studies in this field due to measurement use and invalidity of the BMI scale in a sporting population.

12.3 Obesity Rates in Sport

It is apparent that BMI is not the ideal measure of body composition in sporting athletes and body fat percentage would be far more appropriate. However, despite the above difficulties, one can only use the evidence available to discuss obesity rates in sport and the possible association with increased injury rates.

In the NFL, 56% of players in 2005 were technically obese [23]. In under-20 rugby, 64% of forwards had a BMI >30, considered obese [22]. At the 2003 Rugby World Cup, 25% of players were considered obese [28]. However, even in youth sporting populations, obesity still exists and is a source of ongoing concern. In 9–14 year olds participating in American football, Malina showed 42.6% (38.8–46.5%) of 653 boys to be obese according to the BMI scale [14]. The prevalence of obesity was higher in early maturing players as well as offensive and defensive linemen. This percentage is far greater than the Center for Disease Control's (CDC) estimate of 19.7% of 2–19-year-old Americans being obese [29]. Choate et al. found obesity rates, using BMI percentiles, in 3970 male high school sporting participants to be no different to the general population, although the rates in those who played football and wrestling were higher than that of the general population [13]. Turner reported a reduced obesity prevalence of 16.6% in boys and 15.3% in girls in a 6667 cohort of 12–19-year-old American high school sports participants [30]. Unfortunately, there is a lack of research looking at obesity rates in sub-elite levels of various sports at an adult level to allow for a stronger comparison to be made between elite and sub-elite levels of obesity.

12.4 Obesity as a Risk Factor for Sports Injuries

In recent decades, research in strategies to reduce injury rates has increased exponentially. A plethora of potential risk factors have been identified for various sporting injuries. These risk factors can be both extrinsic and intrinsic. Extrinsic risk factors are those that are external and largely uncontrollable to the athlete. Examples of these include surface, weather and footwear. Intrinsic factors are risk factors that are internal, within the body and are, at least, partially under the athlete's control. These will include age, fitness levels and body mass [31]. A considerable amount of research has been carried out exploring the possibility of a relationship between body mass and injury risk (Table 12.1). Additionally, as obesity rates have risen globally, especially in the Western world, there has been an increased interest in the possible association between obesity and sports injuries.

12.4.1 Evidence for Obesity as a Risk Factor for Sports Injury

Kaplan's study using body mass and skinfolds as body composition measures represents one of the earliest studies in this area [17]. In this study, 98 adolescent American football players were monitored over the course of a single preseason

Table 12.1 Obesity and sports injuries

Author	Aim	Sport	Sample size	Obesity measure	Findings
Kaplan et al. (1995) [20]	To assess relative risk of musculoskeletal injury of obese adolescents' participation in high school football	American football	98 high school players	Body mass and skinfolds	High body mass (>90 kg) was associated with a 2.5× increased injury risk
Lee et al. (1997) [21]	To determine whether there is an association between players' physique and injuries incurred while playing rugby football	Rugby	66 senior club rugby players	BMI and somatotyping	Endomorphs more likely to suffer injury than ectomorphs after age-adjustment
Gómez et al. (1998) [15]	To determine whether associations exist between body fatness and injury rates in high school football linemen	American football	215 high school football linemen	BMI and body fat percentage	Higher BMI was associated with increased lower extremity injury
Bazelmans et al. (2004) [3]	To look at the relationship between obesity and trauma among young people in the Hainaut Province in Belgium	Various	2363 children	BMI and skinfolds	Childhood obesity increases injury occurrence
Tyler et al. (2006) [32]	To examine the association between BMI, a history of previous ankle sprain and risk of sustaining noncontact ankle injury	American football	152 high school players	BMI	High BMI doubled risk of suffering ankle injury
Rose et al. (2008) [11]	To examine the sociodemographic risk factors for sport injury in adolescents	Various	2721 high school athletes	BMI	Students in the 50–90th BMI percentile were most likely to suffer injury

(continued)

Table 12.1 (continued)

Author	Aim	Sport	Sample size	Obesity measure	Findings
Yard and Comstock (2011) [10]	To examine injury patterns by BMI in high school athletes	Various	13,881 injuries across 100 schools	BMI	Obese athletes suffered greater proportion of knee injuries and injuries due to contact with another player
Richmond et al. (2013) [2]	To investigate the relationship between sport injury and BMI in adolescents	Various	4339 high school athletes	BMI	34% increased risk of injury for obese athletes
Nilstad et al. (2014) [12]	To investigate risk factors for lower extremity injuries in elite female soccer players	Soccer	173 elite Norwegian soccer players	BMI	BMI associated with new lower extremity injury
Ridley et al. (2014) [6]	To evaluate the impact of body mass index (BMI) on complications and associated injuries in patients undergoing surgical treatment for multiligamentous knee injuries	Various, general population	126 injuries	BMI	A 1-unit increase in BMI increased the odds ratio of complications by 9.2%
Richmond et al. (2016) [5]	To examine body mass index (BMI) and waist circumference (WC) as risk factors for sport injury in adolescents	Various	1040 adolescents	BMI and waist circumference	Increased risk of time loss injury and knee injury in adolescents that were overweight/obese

block and their results found that a high body mass (>90 kg) was associated with a 2.5× greater risk of suffering an injury. They also showed a significant relationship existed between body weight and injury risk ($p < 0.05$, $r = 0.27$). Gomez et al., in a high school football population, found that a higher BMI, as well as body fatness, was a risk factor for lower extremity injury in 215 linemen [15]. Their results showed a BMI of between 24 and 36 kg/m^2, except at 34 kg/m^2, leaving a lineman at a 1.86–3× increased risk of sustaining an injury to the lower extremity. A 2006 study led by Tyler focused on BMI risk and ankle sprains in high school football players [32]. Their results highlighted a 3.9× increased injury incidence in overweight players compared to normal weight across 1–3 seasons. The authors also noted an overweight player with a history of a previous ankle sprain was 19× more likely to suffer an ankle injury than a player of normal weight with no previous history of ankle injury. A Canadian study by Rose in adolescent sporting participants also found an association between BMI and injury risk [11]. Using BMI percentiles, the authors stated that participants in the 50–90th BMI percentile (23–26 kg/m^2) had the greatest risk of injury among the 2721 adolescents ($p < 0.001$, OR = 1.58, 1.66).

In Richmond's 2013 study of 4339 high school athletes, students classified as obese were 34% more likely to suffer an injury across 1 year (OR = 1.34, 95%CI: 1.02–1.80) [2]. Her 2016 study investigated a smaller population (1040 junior high school students), yet results still showed those in the overweight and obese brackets to have an increased risk of time loss injury (IRR = 2.82, 95%CI: 1.01–8.04) and knee injury (IRR = 2.07, 95%CI: 1.00–6.94) [5]. It was noted, however, that the all injury and lower extremity injury risk increase was not statistically significant. Bazelman's cross-sectional study in a Belgian population of 2363 students showed 15% of the participants to be obese according to World Health Organization (WHO) classifications [3]. In analysing this 15%, the results determined a significantly higher frequency of injury in the obese individuals ($p = 0.003$, 44% versus 36%). Finally, in a youth population, a large study by Yard and Comstock in 2011 gathered information from 100 Certified Athletic Trainers (ATCs) across the United States over 4 years [10]. The ATCs reported 13,881 injuries across the study period. The results found that the prevalence of obese and overweight athletes was the highest in injured American football players (54.4%). Obese athletes also suffered a greater amount of knee injuries compared with their normal-weight counterparts [injury proportion ratio (IPR) = 1.27, 95%CI: 1.14–1.42]. These individuals also presented differing mechanisms of injury with a greater likelihood of sustaining injury via contact with another player (IPR = 1.31, 95%CI: 1.26–1.37). The quantity of research in youth populations is expansive. This could be attributed to the ease of data collection with such large sample sizes available. It could also be theorised that, at adult level, less people with a high BMI participate in sport, relative to an adolescent population. Sport participation is thoroughly encouraged in high school and there are little barriers to participation. The same incentive and ease of participation do not exist at an adult level. Hence, the majority of evidence establishing a relationship between obesity and sports injuries being in an adolescent population may be ascribable to relatively more obese individuals participating in sport at a young level. Similar to obesity rates, a greater emphasis should be placed on investigating this relationship in adult populations.

In saying this, some evidence does exist in other populations, including the elite athlete. In elite female soccer in Norway, a thorough screening was performed on 173 athletes including body composition, strength, balance and biomechanics, and the athletes were tracked across a single season [12]. The only measure that had an association with new lower extremity injury was BMI (OR = 1.51, 95%CI: 1.21–1.90, $p = 0.001$). Based on a multivariate analysis performed, a higher BMI was shown to increase thigh injury risk by 51% per standard deviation (SD). Lee et al. looked into body composition's effect on injury occurrence in senior rugby in Scotland across an entire season [21]. They used somatotyping as a body composition measurement and found, after adjusting for age, that endomorphs (deemed obese) to be more likely than ectomorphs (normal) to sustain an injury in a match ($p < 0.0001$). It is interesting to note that, even at high levels of sport, a relationship appears to exist between obesity and sporting injuries. Further research in different elite and sub-elite populations is warranted.

A review paper by Wilder and Cicchetti covered common injuries with athletes with obesity in great detail [4]. Much of the evidence used in this study is based on a general population and the authors link to potential sporting injuries. The review claimed obese children had lower bone mineral content and would be more susceptible to fractures in a contact sport. Factors such as reduced femoral anteversion, increased Q-angle, mean peak forefoot pressure and flatter feet may be more prevalent in obese children and may negatively impact their sporting participation. Potential mechanisms such as these will be covered later in the chapter in more detail. In a case-control study in runners highlighted in this review, a BMI >30 kg/m^2 was associated with an increased risk of developing plantar fasciitis [33].

Due to its large financial, physical and mental burden, anterior cruciate ligament (ACL) injury has also been a focus of research with regards to body mass [34]. In 118 participants including injured and uninjured individuals, Bojicic et al. looked to quantify the relationship between BMI and knee parameters on ACL injury risk and found that, for every 1-unit BMI increase, when coupled with a 1° posterior tibial slope, the risk of suffering an ACL injury rose by 15% [9]. Other studies also explored this relationship in military populations and, despite not necessarily being a sporting population, ACL injury occurs so frequently in sport that these studies are worth delving into. The first is a 2003 study by Uhorchack, which found women with an above-normal BMI to be at greater risk of suffering a non-contact ACL injury ($p = 0.008$) [7]. Evans also highlighted BMI as being independently associated with ACL injury in 1687 military subjects with injured subjects presenting overweight (25.6 ± 3.6 kg/m^2) and uninjured presenting as normal weight (24.4 ± 2.9 kg/m^2) ($p = 0.005$) [8].

BMI has not only been associated with an increased risk of injury occurrence, but also increased risk of a poor prognosis post-injury. A 2014 study by Ridley et al. focused solely on obesity with regards to multi-ligamentous injury [6]. They investigated the effect of BMI on complications and associated injuries in patients requiring multi-ligamentous surgery, commonly seen in sporting situations. The study took place across 10 years in 123 patients. They found that the rates of surgical complications in obese patients were 15.4% compared to 8.05% in non-obese. The authors were also able to show that a 1-unit increase in BMI increased the likelihood of complications by 9.2% ($p = 0.0174$). No other research in sport-related injuries currently exists evaluating obesity as a risk factor for poor injury prognosis. In theory, decreasing BMI in the post-surgical process may be advantageous with regards to injury prognosis.

12.5 Mechanisms by Which Obesity Is a Risk Factor for Sports Injury

The evidence appears to suggest that obesity is a risk factor for sporting injury. Although the mechanism of injury and how it differs from the general population has not been studied extensively and, as such, the evidence is far from conclusive. Much of the reasoning suggested in the literature is speculative in nature, and this has been noted by the authors of these studies. The aforementioned issues with the BMI scale cause further ambiguity. Judging by the available research, the reasoning behind this potential association is likely multifactorial and not solely attributable to a single factor.

The most frequently suggested mechanism for obesity as a risk factor for sports injury is increased joint loading due to increased body mass. Both Richmond and Nilstad speculated that athletes with a higher BMI are less capable of absorbing sustained forces in sport [2, 12]. Obesity appears to be a risk factor for knee joint injuries in particular [8]. A higher BMI has been associated with increased peak knee compressive and shear forces [35]. Hence, it is plausible to suggest that a higher BMI causes greater joint loading that, either acutely or chronically, the body cannot withstand. It may also accentuate forces placed on the athlete when faced with a biomechanically challenging position such as hyperextension or valgus at the knee. The athlete's increased BMI may increase the force applied and leave the athlete more susceptible to injury than an athlete of lower BMI. This is especially relevant in impact sports, such as American football, Gaelic games, soccer and rugby.

Another mechanism that has been proposed relates to the suggestion that obese individuals may be less physically active and accustomed to high-impact activity [2, 32]. The obesity literature claims that obese people spend less time in moderate to vigorous physical activity than those of normal weight [2]. Most sporting activities will incorporate and be dominated by moderate to vigorous physical activity. Consequently, Tyler postulated that it is the lack of time spent in weight-bearing activity that causes obese individuals to be at an increased risk of injury as they are not accustomed to the demands of the activity [38]. Wilder and Cicchetti also claimed that an increase in physical activity may reduce this injury risk in obese sporting participants [4]. The greater experience one has in a sport, the greater competency they will likely have to cope with the physical demands of the sport and this should leave them at a decreased risk of injury. It must be noted that the intensity of work here is key as the increased physical activity of an individual must be of a moderate to vigorous nature to mirror the demands of sport. This mechanism can only be attributed to non-elite sport, however, as elite athletes with a BMI deemed obese will spend adequate time performing moderate to vigorous activity in their sport.

Decreased neuromuscular control is another potential mechanism that has been proposed in the literature [2, 7]. This is likely influenced greatly by the two factors above. Balance and posture have been shown to be poorer in obese individuals compared to normal-weight individuals [36]. Deforche's study assessed for balance ability in obese individuals on a balance beam and was able to highlight decreased ability in individuals with obesity. In this study, the decreased ability could be seen in a quiet environment with little external stimuli. It is reasonable to suggest this poor control would be accentuated in a loud, sporting environment where external stimuli are plentiful. An obese individual's poor balance is likely a result of their increased weight as well as, perhaps, less physical activity and experience in challenging positions. A lack of adequate motor patterning when a limb is placed in a precarious position under excessive load can result in the musculoskeletal structure, whether it is muscle, tendon, ligament or bone, to fail.

Conceivably, as a result of the above factors, obese individuals may develop maladaptive biomechanical alterations that leave them more susceptible to suffering an injury. In a sporting setting this potential risk factor has not been looked at substantially. In Bojicic's previously mentioned study in the military, for every 1-unit increase BMI combined with a 1° increase in posterior slope, ACL injury risk rose by 15% [9]. In a clinical setting, obesity has been associated with a host of musculoskeletal conditions due to altered biomechanics. Obese individuals are more likely to have overpronation at the foot which is a risk factor for chronic heel pain [4]. Those with a higher BMI are also at a greater risk of developing carpal tunnel syndrome due to altered mechanics at the hand and wrist [4]. It is reasonable to suggest that obese sporting participants have similar altered biomechanics which may leave them at great risk of sustaining acute and/or chronic injuries.

A possibility that cannot be overlooked is that obese athletes may play more frequently in positions that involve more physical contact and high impacts. As in the U20 Six Nations Championship, 64% of forwards were obese whereas none of the backs across the six teams had a BMI >30 [22]. In rugby, forwards are seen to be more involved in static activity such as tackling, rucking, scrums and mauls, whereas the backs perform more high-intensity running of longer distance [37]. Therefore, obese individuals are forced to endure higher impacts and more physical activity. As a consequence, their risk of suffering contact injuries will be higher. There is evidence to back this up as Yard and Comstock found obese athletes to suffer more injury from contact with another player than normal-weighted athletes in high school American football (IPR = 1.31, 95%CI: 1.26–1.37) [10].

A final potential mechanism for obesity as a risk factor for injury is lower fitness levels. Obese individuals are known to have lower aerobic fitness on average than those of normal weight [38]. There is no great evidence to suggest this is a risk factor. However, although speculation, a mechanism can be theorised. If an obese individual were to have less physical fitness, they would likely incur greater fatigue coming towards the end of a training/match. Fatigue has been shown to cause a greater risk of injury [39]. Hence, if an obese individual fatigues quicker than an athlete of normal weight, coupled with their poor neuromuscular control, they will be at a far greater risk of suffering injury.

12.6 Obesity and Injury Patterns

It is important to recognise that the injury pattern in obese individuals appears to differ from that of normal-weighted individuals. Based on the above evidence, lower extremity injuries appear far more prevalent in obese individuals. Yard and Comstock found that obese athletes suffered a greater proportion of knee injuries than normal-weight athletes across high school sports (18.3% versus 14.3%; IPR = 1.27, 95%CI: 1.14–1.42) [10]. Certain sports also showed increased prevalence of injury in obese athletes, also. Obese athletes suffered an increased proportion of ankle/foot injuries in wrestling (15.8% versus 6.4%; IPR = 2.46, 95%CI: 1.56–3.87), volleyball (64.7% versus 37.8%; IPR = 1.71, 95%CI: 1.18–2.49) and football (18.8% versus 16.0%; IPR = 1.18, 95%CI: 1.03–1.35). In football linemen, BMI and higher body fat were correlated with a greater prevalence of lower extremity injury, with BMI showing the strongest association [15]. With regards to ankle injury alone, BMI was claimed to be a risk factor for injury ($p < 0.05$). All evidence currently available appears to suggest that obese individuals are at greater risk of suffering lower extremity injuries. This is likely attributable to the aforementioned increased joint loading an obese individual experiences, especially in the lower extremity [2, 12, 41].

12.7 Effect of Injury on Obesity Development

The potential effect of obesity on sports injury risk has been well defined. However, there is a paucity of information available on the inverse of this relationship; the effect of sports injury on the risk of becoming obese. Following injury, a period of rehabilitation is almost always required. This often causes a reduction in physical activity and energy expenditure [9]. Over 6 months after ACL reconstruction, moderate to vigorous physical activity is seen to reduce by 14 min/day and step count decreasing by 1611 steps/day [40]. This has been linked with weight gain and increase in obesity markers [9]. In a female sporting population, knee injury suffered in their adolescent years was associated with increased BMI ($p = 0.03$) and body fat percentage scores ($p = 0.009$) after 1 year [41]. As noted by de Oliveira and colleagues, little is known about the long-term effects of injury on obesity [34]. It is often said that an athlete dies twice; once when they take their last breath, and the other when they retire. The effects of participating in elite sport to the body is often life changing, increasing the risk of chronic, long-term disability which can reduce mobility in later life increasing the likelihood of weight gain. However, the psychological effect of retirement is also quite profound, with a high percentage of athletes suffering depression (4–29%) after their careers have ended [42, 43]. This can also increase the risk of obesity and these previously heralded individuals can indeed become quite vulnerable when the crowds stop cheering [16, 44].

12.8 Summary

In conclusion, a relationship appears to exist between obesity and sports injury. It is clear that the definition of obesity is not fit for purpose with regards to the use of the BMI scale. The obesity rates in sports are population and sport dependent but across all ages and sports, obesity does exist. It is plausible to suggest that, despite methodological difficulties with regards to BMI, these individuals, particularly in a non-elite environment, may be at a greater risk of suffering injury. The evidence for this appears strong in young, adolescent populations. Obese sporting individuals may also be at an increased risk of suffering lower limb injuries, in particular, due to the injury patterns that obese individuals present with in sport. Additionally, obesity may leave an athlete requiring surgical intervention more susceptible to complications and poorer prognosis post-surgery. Inversely, athletes who suffer injuries, particularly of a long-term nature, may be predisposed to developing obesity. Sport offers a plethora of physical, mental and emotional benefits for all individuals across all populations. Injury, however, is part and parcel of sport and cannot be prevented in its entirety. Certain sports and certain intrinsic factors will have a greater risk of injury and obesity is likely one of these factors.

References

1. Anandacoomarasamy A, Caterson I, Sambrook P, Fransen M, March L. The impact of obesity on the musculoskeletal system. Int J Obes. 2008;32(2):211–22.
2. Richmond SA, Kang J, Emery CA. Is body mass index a risk factor for sport injury in adolescents? J Sci Med Sport. 2013;16(5):401–5.
3. Bazelmans C, Coppieters Y, Godin I, Parent F, Berghmans L, Dramaix M, et al. Is obesity associated with injuries among young people? Eur J Epidemiol. 2004;19(11):1037–42.
4. Wilder RP, Cicchetti M. Common injuries in athletes with obesity and diabetes. Clin Sports Med. 2009;28(3):441–53.
5. Richmond SA, Nettel-Aguirre A, Doyle-Baker PK, Macpherson A, Emery CA. Examining measures of weight as risk factors for sport-related injury in adolescents. J Sports Med. 2016;2016:e7316947.
6. Ridley TJ, Cook S, Bollier M, McCarthy M, Gao Y, Wolf B, et al. Effect of body mass index on patients with multiligamentous knee injuries. Arthroscopy. 2014;30(11):1447–52.
7. Uhorchak JM, Scoville CR, Williams GN, Arciero RA, Pierre PSt, Taylor DC. Risk factors associated with noncontact injury of the anterior cruciate ligament. Am J Sports Med. 2003;31(6):831–42.
8. Evans DC, Stawicki SPA, Davido HT, Eiferman D. Obesity in trauma patients: correlations of body mass index with outcomes, injury patterns, and complications. Am Surg. 2011;77(8):1003–8.
9. Bojicic KM, Beaulieu ML, Imaizumi Krieger DY, Ashton-Miller JA, Wojtys EM. Association between lateral posterior tibial slope, body mass index, and ACL injury risk. Orthop J Sports Med. 2017;5(2) https://doi.org/10.1177/2325967116688664.

10. Yard E, Comstock D. Injury patterns by body mass index in US high school athletes. J Phys Act Health. 2011;8(2):182–91. https://doi.org/10.1123/jpah.8.2.182.
11. Rose MS, Emery CA, Meeuwisse WH. Sociodemographic predictors of sport injury in adolescents. Med Sci Sports Exerc. 2008;40(3):444–50.
12. Nilstad A, Andersen TE, Bahr R, Holme I, Steffen K. Risk factors for lower extremity injuries in elite female soccer players. Am J Sports Med. 2014;42(4):940–8.
13. Choate N, Forster C, Almquist J, Olsen C, Poth M. The prevalence of overweight in participants in high school extramural sports. J Adolesc Health. 2007;40(3):283–5.
14. Malina RM, Morano PJ, Barron M, Miller SJ, Cumming SP, Kontos AP, et al. Overweight and obesity among youth participants in American football. J Pediatr. 2007;151(4):378–82.
15. Gómez JE, Ross SK, Calmbach WL, Kimmel RB, Schmidt DR, Dhanda R. Body fatness and increased injury rates in high school football linemen. Clin J Sport Med. 1998;8(2):115–20.
16. Emami M, Behforouz A, Jarahi L, Zarifian A, Rashidlamir A, Rashed MM, et al. The risk of developing obesity, insulin resistance, and metabolic syndrome in former power-sports athletes—does sports career termination increase the risk. Indian J Endocrinol Metab. 2018;22(4):515–9.
17. Nuttall FQ. Body mass index. Nutr Today. 2015;50(3):117–28.
18. Physical status: the use and interpretation of anthropometry. Report of a WHO Expert Committee. World Health Organ Tech Rep Ser. 1995;854:1–452.
19. Smalley KJ, Knerr AN, Kendrick ZV, Colliver JA, Owen OE. Reassessment of body mass indices. Am J Clin Nutr. 1990;52(3):405–8.
20. Kaplan TA, Digel SL, Scavo VA, Arellana SB. Effect of obesity on injury risk in high school football players. Clin J Sport Med. 1995;5(1):43–7.
21. Lee AJ, Myers JL, Garraway WM. Influence of players' physique on rugby football injuries. Br J Sports Med. 1997;31(2):135–8. [cited 2023 Jun 6]. Available from: https://www.ncbi.nlm.nih.gov/pmc/articles/PMC1332613/.
22. Fennell W. Six nations under age rugby and BMI, what price success? Heart. 2022;108(Suppl 3):A56.
23. Harp JB, Hecht L. Obesity in the National Football League. JAMA. 2005;293(9):1061–2.
24. Gavarry O, Lentin G, Pezery P, Delextrat A, Chaumet G, Boussuges A, et al. A cross-sectional study assessing the contributions of body fat mass and fat-free mass to body mass index scores in male youth rugby players. Sports Med Open. 2018;4(1):17.
25. Pontaga I, Zidens J. Estimation of body mass index in team sports athletes. Lase J Sport Sci. 2011;2(2):33–44.
26. Lombard AJJ. Strength and energetics of elite rugby union players. Afr J Phys Act Health Sci. 2003;9(3):89–99.
27. VO2 Max: The Fitness Metric That Can Help You Run Faster and Work Out Harder [Internet]. CNET. [cited 2023 Jun 6]. Available from: https://www.cnet.com/health/fitness/vo2-max-the-fitness-metric-that-can-help-you-run-faster-and-workout-harder/.
28. King NA, Hills AP, Blundell JE. High body mass index is not a barrier to physical activity: analysis of international rugby players' anthropometric data. Eur J Sport Sci. 2005;5(2):73–5.
29. Childhood Obesity Facts | Overweight & Obesity | CDC [Internet] 2022. [cited 2023 Jun 8]. Available from: https://www.cdc.gov/obesity/data/childhood.html.
30. Turner RW, Perrin EM, Coyne-Beasley T, Peterson CJ, Skinner AC. Reported sports participation, race, sex, ethnicity, and obesity in US adolescents from NHANES physical activity (PAQ_D). Glob Pediatr Health. 2015;2:2333794X15577944.
31. Wang V, Mayer F, Bonaventura K, Wippert M. Intrinsic and extrinsic injury risk factors of elite winter sports athlete in training. Br J Sports Med. 2017;51(4):406.
32. Tyler TF, McHugh MP, Mirabella MR, Mullaney MJ, Nicholas SJ. Risk factors for noncontact ankle sprains in high school football players: the role of previous ankle sprains and body mass index. Am J Sports Med. 2006;34(3):471–5.
33. Riddle DL, Pulisic M, Pidcoe P, Johnson RE. Risk factors for Plantar fasciitis: a matched case-control study. J Bone Joint Surg Am. 2003;85(5):872–7.

34. de Oliveira FCL, Roy JS, Pappas E. ACL injury, physical activity, and overweight/obesity: a vicious cycle? Knee Surg Sports Traumatol Arthrosc. 2020;28(3):667–9.
35. Messier SP, Pater M, Beavers DP, Legault C, Loeser RF, Hunter DJ, et al. Influences of alignment and obesity on knee joint loading in osteoarthritic gait. Osteoarthr Cartil. 2014;22(7):912–7.
36. Deforche B, Hills A, Worringham C, PsW D, Murphy AJ, Bouckaert J, et al. Balance and postural skills in normal-weight and overweight prepubertal boys. Int J Pediatr Obes. IJPO Off J Int Assoc Study Obes. 2009;4:175–82.
37. La Monica MB, Fukuda DH, Miramonti AA, Beyer KS, Hoffman MW, Boone CH, et al. Physical differences between forwards and backs in American collegiate rugby players. J Strength Cond Res. 2016;30(9):2382.
38. Ding C, Jiang Y. The relationship between body mass index and physical fitness among Chinese university students: results of a longitudinal study. Healthcare. 2020;8(4):570.
39. Verschueren J, Tassignon B, De Pauw K, Proost M, Teugels A, Van Cutsem J, et al. Does acute fatigue negatively affect intrinsic risk factors of the lower extremity injury risk profile? A systematic and critical review. Sports Med Auckl NZ. 2020;50(4):767–84.
40. Bell DR, Pfeiffer KA, Cadmus-Bertram LA, Trigsted SM, Kelly A, Post EG, et al. Objectively measured physical activity in patients after anterior cruciate ligament reconstruction. Am J Sports Med. 2017;45(8):1893–900.
41. Myer GD, Faigenbaum AD, Foss KB, Xu Y, Khoury J, Dolan LM, et al. Injury initiates unfavourable weight gain and obesity markers in youth. Br J Sports Med. 2014;48(20):1477–81.
42. Mannes ZL, Waxenberg LB, Cottler LB, Perlstein WM, Burrell LE, Ferguson EG, et al. Prevalence and correlates of psychological distress among retired elite athletes: a systematic review. Int Rev Sport Exerc Psychol. 2019;12(1):265–94.
43. Esopenko C, Coury JR, Pieroth EM, Noble JM, Trofa DP, Bottiglieri TS. The psychological burden of retirement from sport. Curr Sports Med Rep. 2020;19(10):430–7.
44. Altowerqi Z, Zainuddin Z, Mohd Hashim AH, Almarwaey A. Are former athletes protected against obesity after retirement? Indian J Public Health Res Dev. 2020;11:1989.

13 Preoperative and Perioperative Anaesthesia in Obesity

Aoife Brady and Alan Gaffney

13.1 Introduction

The prevalence of obesity in the community and, therefore, the number of patients with obesity presenting for musculoskeletal surgery are increasing over time. The safe management of patients with obesity presents many challenges to the multidisciplinary team (MDT), including the anaesthesiologist. The type and degree of obesity, associated comorbidities and their severity, and the type and duration of surgery all impact perioperative risk. The aim of this chapter is to aid the anaesthesiologist in assessing, mitigating and managing risk to optimise the outcome for this important patient group.

13.2 Preoperative Assessment

Ideally, patients with obesity scheduled for surgery should be assessed by a preoperative MDT. There should be a robust referral process to other specialist services (e.g. cardiology, endocrinology) and for further investigations (e.g. echocardiography, sleep studies). The National Confidential Enquiry into Patient Outcome and Death (NCEPOD) review of the perioperative care of surgical patients found that high-risk patients undergoing elective surgery who did not attend a pre-assessment clinic had a 30-day mortality almost 7 times greater than those who did attend (4.8% vs. 0.7%) [1].

A. Brady (✉)
University Hospital Waterford, Waterford, Ireland

A. Gaffney
Beaumont Hospital, Dublin, Ireland
e-mail: Alangaffney@beaumont.ie

J. M. O´Byrne et al. (eds.), *Musculoskeletal Disease and Obesity*,
https://doi.org/10.1007/978-3-031-63310-2_13

A detailed medical, surgical and anaesthetic history should be obtained and physical examination, including a thorough airway assessment, should be performed. Height and weight should be accurately measured and lean body and adjusted body weight should be calculated. All measurements should be clearly documented. History and examination should aim to elicit signs of secondary obesity-related physical attributes. Additional speciality referral and investigations should be guided by history and examination findings.

There are a number of obesity-specific red flags that should prompt further investigation. These are listed in Table 13.1.

13.2.1 Comorbidities Associated with Obesity

Patients with obesity and comorbidities associated with obesity present a higher perioperative risk than those with obesity alone. Common comorbidities associated with obesity are detailed in Table 13.2.

13.2.1.1 Sleep-Disordered Breathing

Sleep-disordered breathing, including obstructive sleep apnoea (OSA) and obesity hypoventilation syndrome (OHS), is of particular concern. Sleep-disordered breathing can lead to pulmonary hypertension, heart failure, chronic hypoxaemia and hypercapnia. Patients with these conditions are at an increased risk for difficult airway management, oxygen desaturation, respiratory failure, need for postoperative reintubation of the trachea and postoperative cardiopulmonary complications. If diagnosed and treated preoperatively with nighttime continuous positive airway

Table 13.1 Red flags [2]

Red flags	Comment
Poor functional capacity	MET <4
Abnormal ECG	For example, heart strain, axis deviation, ischaemia, ventricular hypertrophy
Uncontrolled hypertension, heart failure or ischaemic heart disease	Specialist investigations and cardiology referral may be required
SpO_2 <94% on room air	May indicate sleep-disordered breathing
Bicarbonate >28 mmol/L	May indicate sleep-disordered breathing
History of thromboembolic disease	Increased risk of perioperative thromboembolic disease
STOP-BANG questionnaire score greater ≥6	High risk of sleep-disordered breathing
Metabolic syndrome	Three or more of hypertension, insulin resistance, impaired glucose tolerance, decreased serum high-density lipoprotein (HDL), increased serum triglycerides and large waist circumference

MET metabolic equivalent task, *ECG* electrocardiogram, *ECHO* echocardiogram, SpO_2 peripheral oxygen saturation, *STOP-BANG* obstructive sleep apnoea risk score

Table 13.2 Comorbidities associated with obesity

Sleep-disordered breathing
Asthma
Hypertension
Left ventricular hypertrophy or failure
Right-sided heart failure
Cardiac conduction abnormalities
Cardiomyopathy
Metabolic syndrome
Diabetes mellitus
Reduced functional capacity
Venous thromboembolism
Non-alcoholic fatty liver disease

Table 13.3 STOP-BANG questionnaire and interpretation

Question/observation	1 point if the following
Do you snore loudly?	Yes
Do you often feel tired, fatigued or sleepy during the daytime?	Yes
Has anyone observed you stop breathing?	Yes
Do you have high blood pressure?	Yes
BMI	≥35 kg/m^2
Age	>50
Neck circumference	>40 cm
Gender	Male

Interpretation of score:

- 0–2: Low risk for moderate-to-severe OSA
- 3–5: Intermediate risk for moderate-to-severe OSA
- 6–8: High risk for moderate-to-severe OSA

pressure (CPAP), the risk of complications is reduced [3]. Therefore, where suspected, patients with these conditions should be referred preoperatively for sleep studies and assessment by a respiratory specialist.

The STOP-BANG scoring system is used to screen for possible sleep-disordered breathing (Table 13.3).

Patients can be further screened for risk of OSA using STOP-BANG tool and further parameters as described in Table 13.4. All patients who are deemed high risk for OSA from OSA screening should be referred for sleep studies and assessed by a respiratory specialist prior to surgery.

The degree of risk for sleep-disordered breathing can help predict the level of postoperative care required. The most suitable management and location of postoperative care for patients depending on OSA risk are suggested in Table 13.5.

13.2.1.2 Cardiovascular Disease

Patients with obesity have an increased cardiac workload and are at an increased risk of hypertension, arrhythmias (sino-atrial node dysfunction and fatty infiltration of the conducting system), left ventricular hypertrophy, QT prolongation, ischaemic heart disease and heart failure.

Table 13.4 OSA screening algorithm for patients with obesity [2]

Low risk	Moderate risk	High risk
STOP-BANG 0–2 and ASA 1 or 2	STOP-BANG 0–2 + ASA 3 or greater + no further risk factors	STOP-BANG 0–2 + ASA 3 or greater + further risk factors
	STOP-BANG 3–5 + any ASA + no further risk factors	STOP-BANG 3–5 + any ASA grade + further risk factors
		STOP-BANG 6–8

Further risk factors:

- Mallampati score 3–4
- Neck circumference >50 cm
- SpO_2 <94%
- Bicarbonate >28
- New York Heart Association Functional classification grade III or more

Table 13.5 Postoperative management algorithm for patients with obesity according to OSA risk [2]

Level of post-op care	Ward	Low opioid + SpO_2 monitoring overnight	Invasive monitoring + HDU
Criteria	Low risk OSA screening + easy airway	Low risk OSA screening + not easy airway	Proven OSA not well established on CPAP, e.g., no clinical improvement or non-compliant
		Moderate risk OSA screening	
		Mild/moderate proven OSA not requiring CPAP	High risk for OSA on screening that has not undergone sleep studies
		Proven OSA well managed on CPAP (compliant and clinical benefit)	Proven OSA well managed on CPAP (compliant and clinical benefit) likely to require very high dose opioids

History and examination should aim to elicit signs and symptoms of cardiac dysfunction such as exertional chest pain, exertional shortness of breath, cardiac syncope, orthopnoea, paroxysmal nocturnal dyspnoea, oedema, hypertension, murmurs or added heart sounds or a reduction in exercise tolerance.

Exercise tolerance is estimated using the metabolic equivalent of task (MET) score (Table 13.6). Patients are generally considered metabolically fit for surgery when the MET score is 4 or more.

Preoperative ECG should be performed in patients with obesity with signs or symptoms of cardiac pathology. ECG changes could include heart strain, axis deviation, ischaemia or ventricular hypertrophy. ECHO should be performed if there are signs or symptoms of structural or functional disease. Referral to a cardiologist for preoperative review and further cardiac work-up should be considered in patients with positive investigations or concerning cardiac signs and symptoms.

Table 13.6 MET score

MET score	Activity examples
1	Sitting watching television
2	Light gardening, getting dressed, showering, walking down steps
3	Housework, walking on the flat
4	Walking up a flight of stairs
5	Social dancing, walking 6 km/h
6	9 holes golf carrying clubs, using a push mower
7	Hiking, singles tennis, heavy gardening
8	Slow jogging, moving heavy furniture
9	Cycling at moderate pace, slow skipping
>10	Strenuous sports

13.2.1.3 Metabolic Syndrome

Metabolic syndrome is a group of symptoms that include three or more of hypertension, insulin resistance, impaired glucose tolerance, decreased serum high-density lipoprotein (HDL), increased serum triglycerides and large waist circumference. Metabolic syndrome is associated with an increased risk of heart disease, stroke and type 2 diabetes mellitus.

13.2.2 Risk Assessment

Perioperative scores such as the American Society of Anesthesiologists (ASA) score, the Obesity Surgery Mortality Risk Score (OS-MRS), the Surgical Outcome Risk Tool (SORT) score and the American College of Surgeons National Surgical Quality Improvement Program (ACS NSQIP) surgical risk calculator can help to more objectively predict perioperative risk.

A 'high-risk' surgical patient is defined as having a predicted hospital mortality of greater than or equal to 5% [4].

Obesity is divided by increasing body mass index (BMI) into three classes: class 1 obesity (BMI 30–34.9 kg/m^2), class 2 obesity (BMI 35–39.9 kg/m^2) and class 3 obesity (BMI >40 kg/m^2).

The distribution of adipose tissue may, however, be more accurate in predicting perioperative risk than BMI. Central obesity (a waist circumference >102 cm in men and > 88 cm in women) is associated with an increased risk of overall perioperative risk [5]. In particular, there is an increased prevalence of metabolic syndrome, cardiovascular disease and difficulty with airway management and lung ventilation in patients with central obesity [2].

13.2.2.1 ASA Grade

Preoperative physical status is classified by the American Society of Anaesthesiologists (ASA) on a scale of increasing comorbidity from grade 1 to grade 5 (Table 13.7). Used alongside other factors such as the type of surgery, it can be used to help predict perioperative risks [6]. Where a patient has obesity alone, with no additional comorbidities and all else being equal, a patient with class 1 obesity is considered ASA grade 1, a patient with class 2 obesity is ASA grade 2 and a patient with class 3 obesity is ASA grade 3.

For patients with class 3 obesity, perioperative morbidity and mortality are increased. On the other hand, patients with class 1 and 2 obesity have lower rates of morbidity and mortality compared to non-obese patients, all else being equal. This phenomenon is not fully understood and is known as the 'obesity paradox' [7].

13.2.2.2 OS-MRS Score

The Obesity Surgery Mortality Risk Score (OS-MRS) was developed to understand the risk of postoperative mortality in patients undergoing bariatric surgery. It is, however, often used in practice for patients with obesity undergoing other surgical procedures [8]. Table 13.8 outlines the OS-MRS score.

Table 13.7 ASA score

ASA score	Definition	Adult examples
1	Normal healthy patient	Healthy, non-smoker, no or minimal alcohol use
2	Mild systemic disease	Mild diseases without functional limitations—smoker, social alcohol drinker, obesity (BMI 30–40), well-controlled hypertension or diabetes mellitus, mild lung disease
3	Severe systemic disease	Functional limitations—poorly controlled hypertension or diabetes mellitus, COPD, class 3 obesity (BMI > 40), active hepatitis, alcohol dependence or abuse, pacemaker, moderate reduction of ejection fraction, end-stage kidney disease (ESKD) undergoing regular dialysis, myocardial infarction/cerebrovascular accident/transient ischaemic attack/cardiac stents greater than 3 months ago
4	Severe systemic disease that is a constant threat to life	Myocardial infarction/cerebrovascular accident/transient ischaemic attack/cardiac stents less than 3 months ago, ongoing cardiac ischaemia, severe valve dysfunction, severe reduction of ejection fraction, shock, sepsis, disseminated intravascular coagulation, acute respiratory distress syndrome, ESKD not undergoing regular dialysis
5	Moribund, not expected to survive without surgery	Ruptured abdominal/thoracic aneurysm, massive trauma, intracranial bleed with mass effect, ischaemic bowel with multiorgan dysfunction
6	Brain dead patients whose organs are being donated	

Table 13.8 OS-MRS score

Risk factors	Points
Hypertension	1
Age >45	1
Male	1
BMI >50	1
Risk factors for pulmonary thromboembolism: – Previous history pulmonary embolism (PE) or deep vein thrombosis (DVT) – Hypoventilation $PaCO_2$ >45 mmHg – Pulmonary hypertension – Inferior vena cava filter	1

Score	Risk	Mortality (%)
0–1	Low	0.31
2–3	Intermediate	1.9
4–5	High	7.56

13.2.2.3 SORT Score

The Surgical Risk Outcome Tool (SORT) is a tool that predicts the risk of death within 30 days of inpatient surgery [9]. It looks at the type, severity and urgency of the surgical procedure, the patients' ASA score, whether the patient has cancer or not, the patients' age and senior clinicians' clinical risk assessment. It is readily available online and in the app store.

13.2.2.4 ACS NSQIP Surgical Risk Calculator

The risk calculator uses 20 patient predictors and the planned procedure to calculate the risk of 18 specific outcomes within 30 days of the surgery [10]. The calculator can be readily accessed online. Results can be printed and discussed with or given to the patient.

13.2.3 Preoperative Optimisation

Ideally, patients should undergo a programme of preoperative physical optimisation. This may include speciality endocrinology referral for poorly controlled diabetes, cardiology referral where heart failure is poorly controlled or respiratory referral if signs of sleep-disordered breathing or poorly controlled asthma are present.

A preoperative weight loss programme prior to surgery may be considered for patients with class 3 obesity and/or comorbidities associated with obesity. There is no clear evidence, however, that weight loss before orthopaedic surgery definitively improves outcomes although there is some evidence that modest weight loss improves outcomes in bariatric surgery and that bariatric surgery may actually cure knee osteoarthritis symptoms [11–13]. The risks of deferring surgery while undergoing a weight loss programme should be weighed up on an individual basis. The impact of newer weight loss drugs such as semaglutide in the perioperative period is, as yet, unknown [14].

Patients with obesity should be enrolled in the usual enhanced recovery programmes specific to musculoskeletal surgery. The perioperative plan should be clearly explained to patients including medication management, importance of early mobilisation and thromboprophylaxis treatment and a reminder to bring CPAP/BiPAP machines to hospital. Patients should be encouraged and motivated to actively participate in their recovery process and adopt a positive mindset.

13.2.4 Day Case Surgery

Most patients with class 1 and 2 obesity can safely undergo day case surgery if the appropriate resources and trained clinical staff are present [15]. A BMI >40 is not an absolute contraindication for day case surgery but there is an increased risk of perioperative morbidity and mortality in this group, so decisions regarding such patients should be made on a case-by-case basis. Patients with obesity are generally not suitable for day case surgery if significant comorbidities or red flag symptoms as outlined above exist. However, patients with known OSA can undergo day case surgery if they are established on CPAP, have the ability to use it in the postoperative period and where analgesia is expected to be largely non-opioid based [16].

13.3 Intraoperative

13.3.1 Special Planning

Preoperative planning is necessary to ensure that suitable resources are available on the day of surgery. Specialised equipment may be needed (Table 13.9). Additional staff members may be required, such as portering staff, for patient positioning. Risk of injury to staff should be prevented by employing appropriate ergonomics to prevent unnecessary movement of patients. Examples include anaesthetic induction and emergence on the operating table, allowing the patient to self-position on the operating table prior to anaesthesia and moving themselves from the operating table to the bed once surgery is completed. Interestingly, there have been reports of awake intubation with subsequent self-positioning to reduce the likelihood of pressure damage prior to induction of general anaesthesia [17, 18]. Additional time should be allocated for surgical patient positioning.

Pressure points should be carefully padded and protected. Protection of vulnerable nerves with additional padding has been shown to reduce the incidence of intraoperative nerve injury [19]. Rhabdomyolysis has been reported intraoperatively in patients with obesity.

Where possible, the ramped position should be maintained throughout the surgical procedure. Reverse Trendelenburg position may improve pulmonary function compared to the supine position, and certainly compared to the Trendelenberg position [20, 21]. This can be explained by the alleviation of abdominal pressure

Table 13.9 Additional equipment

Blood pressure monitoring: finger cuffs, forearm cuffs, intra-arterial monitoring, large upper arm and calf blood pressure cuffs—size according to manufacturer's instructions
Long epidural/spinal/regional block needles
Large calf compressors and thromboembolic compression stockings
Difficult airway trolley
Additional padding
Slide sheet and/or hoover mattress
Wide Velcro straps and shoulder blocks
Weight-appropriate operating table
Extensions for bed
Ramping pillow
Ultrasound machine
Extra personnel
Large tourniquets
Depth of anaesthesia monitor
Neuromuscular monitor

effects on the diaphragm with the resultant reduction in lung volume, increase in atelectasis and the development of hypoxaemia and postoperative respiratory complications. Prone or lateral positioning may increase the risk of pressure injuries. Lateral positioning is less likely to lead to decreased lung compliance secondary to compression of the dependent lung seen in non-obese patients. This may be due to pressure off-loading of abdominal contents from the diaphragm and lungs [17]. The prone position may improve respiratory function in patients with obesity but comes with risks in the positioning process [17]. Access to the airway in the lateral or prone positioning can be problematic. Should the airway device dislodge, it may be difficult to reposition the patient for reintubation and maintain a patent airway in the meantime.

Intravenous access can occasionally be challenging and may require ultrasound guidance or even central venous access [22].

Blood pressure monitoring can be challenging in patients with obesity. Traditional non-invasive monitoring using arm oscillometry cuffs can be difficult to size and readings may not be accurate. Invasive blood pressure monitoring may be necessary. In a recent study of non-invasive blood pressure monitoring in patients with obesity, finger cuffs were found to be the most accurate followed by forearm oscillometry and lastly arm or lower leg oscillometry [23].

13.3.2 Sedation

Patients with obesity with sleep-disordered breathing are at risk of airway obstruction with procedural sedation. The lowest dose for clinical effect should be administered.

13.3.3 Regional Anaesthesia

Regional anaesthesia includes spinal anaesthesia, epidural anaesthesia and peripheral nerve blocks. Regional anaesthesia offers many intraoperative and postoperative benefits in patients with obesity. Regional anaesthesia for high-risk patients is often preferred as it can avoid general anaesthesia with the requirement for airway manipulation and general anaesthesia-related cardiovascular depression [22]. Regional anaesthesia is associated with a lower risk of VTE than general anaesthesia [24]. Regional anaesthesia can also be opioid-sparing.

Patients with obesity are at an increased risk of opioid-related respiratory depression and airway obstruction, particularly the group that have sleep-disordered breathing. This group is at risk of perioperative hypoventilation and, in the most severe case, respiratory arrest.

Performance of regional anaesthesia procedures can be technically challenging. Landmark techniques are largely impossible, so ultrasound guidance is often required [25]. Ultrasound can aid in the location of the patient's midline, help identify the correct intervertebral space and used to measure the distance from the skin to the epidural or intrathecal space. Longer needles may be needed. The most common length of spinal or epidural needles is 80–90 mm. For patients with obesity, a 120-mm-length needle may be required. Performance of regional anaesthesia may take longer and may require more attempts. Patients with obesity are at a higher risk of block failure [26]. Local anaesthetic agents should be dosed according to lean body weight. Central neuraxial dosing is based on height.

Intrathecal opioids can be used to reduce postoperative opioid requirements in patients with obesity [22, 27, 28]. Consideration should be given for the use of intrathecal morphine in patients where it is expected that substantial doses of systemic postoperative opioid analgesia will be required. However, intrathecal morphine >300 mcg has been associated with respiratory depression [28]. If intrathecal morphine is used, adequate postoperative monitoring for at least 24 h should be arranged. Patients with sleep-disordered breathing should be monitored with continuous pulse oximetry, potentially in an HDU setting. Intrathecal opiates are not suitable for day case surgery [29].

13.3.4 General Anaesthesia

13.3.4.1 Airway and Induction

Patients with obesity are twice as likely to experience adverse airway events compared to patients who do not have obesity [30]. These patients are at an increased risk of difficult bag-mask ventilation and intubation, aspiration and airway obstruction during emergence. In addition, patients are at an increased risk of unsuccessful airway rescue with supraglottic airway devices or cricothyroidotomy. Patients with obesity desaturate more quickly due to increased oxygen consumption, increased work of breathing, reduced chest wall compliance and reduced functional residual capacity. General anaesthesia further reduces functional residual capacity to below closing capacity, resulting in atelectasis. Atelectasis results in shunt and ventilation-perfusion mismatch whereby alveoli are perfused but not ventilated, ultimately leading to desaturation and type 1 respiratory failure.

Tracheal intubation is generally recommended. Patients with obesity are at an increased risk of adverse airway events with the use of supraglottic airways such as aspiration pneumonitis [30]. Difficult airway equipment should be readily available and an airway management plan should be in place prior to induction. Supraglottic airway devices should only be used in carefully selected patients, usually with BMI <40, undergoing short procedures with senior anaesthesiologist involvement [22]. Second-generation supraglottic devices are recommended. The size of an airway device should be selected based on ideal body weight rather than actual weight.

Adequate preoxygenation prior to induction of anaesthesia is important to prevent oxygen desaturation. End-tidal oxygen of at least 80% should be achieved prior to induction. Apnoeic oxygenation using high-flow nasal oxygenation reduces desaturation risk [31].

Induction of anaesthesia should be performed in the ramped position with the tragus of the ear level with the sternal notch. This makes bag-mask ventilation and laryngoscopy easier and increases functional residual capacity. The ramped position aids in laryngoscope insertion by preventing handle obstruction by the chest wall and improving the laryngeal view.

13.3.4.2 Awareness

Patients with obesity are three times more likely to experience awareness under general anaesthesia compared to the general population [32]. This is largely due to the rapid redistribution of intravenous anaesthesia drugs [32]. Anaesthesiologists should be aware of this during induction and maintenance and should potentially consider the depth of anaesthesia monitoring.

13.3.4.3 Drug Dosing

Dosing of drugs in patients with obesity is a complex and understudied area. Basing drug dosing on total body weight can result in overdose and does not take into account the large volume of distribution and the metabolic activity of adipose tissue. Lean body weight (LBW) is generally the most appropriate dosing method for the majority of drugs used during anaesthesia [33]. In certain circumstances, adjusted body weight (ABW) or total body weight (TBW) is used. Many drugs have not been adequately studied in patients with obesity. Table 13.10 outlines suggested weight-based drug dosing for commonly used anaesthetic agents.

13.3.4.4 Maintenance

Either inhalational anaesthesia or total intravenous anaesthesia (TIVA) is appropriate for maintenance of anaesthesia. The pharmacokinetic models for TIVA with propofol, however, have not been validated in patients with obesity. Therefore, the use of depth of anaesthesia monitoring should be considered. Short-acting inhalational volatile agents with a low blood:gas partition coefficient, such as sevoflurane, allow for a rapid onset and offset of action, reduce absorption into adipose tissue and decrease the potential for prolonged emergence from anaesthesia.

Table 13.10 Suggested weight-based drug dose adjustment

LBW	ABW	TBW
Propofol—induction Thiopentone Fentanyl Remifentanil Alfentanil Morphine Atracurium Rocuronium Vecuronium Morphine Paracetamol Local anaesthetics	Propofol—infusion Antibiotics Neostigmine Sugammadex	Suxamethonium Low-molecular-weight heparin

13.3.4.5 Ventilation

Ventilation intraoperatively should follow a lung-protective ventilatory strategy with tidal volumes of 6-8 ml/kg of ideal body weight, appropriate positive end expiratory pressure (PEEP) and low driving pressures (airway plateau pressure minus PEEP) [34, 35]. Lung-protective ventilation strategy has been shown to reduce mortality and ventilator days in patients with acute lung injury and acute respiratory distress syndrome and, thus, is widely adopted during intraoperative ventilation [36]. PEEP should be individualised and titrated to clinical effect, which is generally much higher than required in non-obese patients. This helps splint open the alveoli during expiration by improving the transalveolar pressure gradient and counteracting the excess pressure of the chest wall and abdominal contents, thus preventing alveolar collapse and potentially postoperative respiratory complications. The ramped position should be maintained intraoperatively where possible to help prevent atelectasis. Use of volume control ventilation with high PEEP and a single recruitment manoeuvre in patients with obesity has been associated with improved oxygenation, pulmonary compliance and a reduction in intraoperative atelectasis [35].

13.3.4.6 Neuromuscular Monitoring

Neuromuscular blocking agents should be fully reversed prior to extubation as measured by quantitative and qualitative neuromuscular monitoring, that is, four twitches present in train of four (TOF) count and a TOF ratio of 0.9 or greater [22]. Sugammadex is the preferred reversal agent in patients where rocuronium or vecuronium has been used [37]. Wide-awake extubation in the ramped position is ideal. Airway reflexes should have returned and patients should be spontaneously ventilating with adequate tidal volumes and a regular respiratory pattern. Preemptive nasopharyngeal airway placement can be useful to manage potential postoperative airway obstruction.

13.3.5 Venous Thromboembolism (VTE) Prophylaxis

Patients with obesity are at an increased risk of venous thromboembolism [38]. All patients should be risk assessed for VTE on admission to hospital. All patients should receive pharmacological prophylaxis and wear thromboembolic deterrent stockings unless there is a specific contraindication. Intraoperative use of intermittent pneumatic compression devices should be used where possible. Regional anaesthesia carries a lower risk of VTE compared to general anaesthesia.

13.3.6 Multimodal Analgesia

Multimodal analgesia reduces opioid requirements. Paracetamol and non-steroidal anti-inflammatory drugs (NSAIDs) should be considered where there are no contraindications. Analgesic adjuncts such as regional anaesthesia and intravenous lidocaine, clonidine, ketamine and magnesium should be considered. If opioids are required, short-acting agents are preferred. Avoid the concurrent use of long-acting sedative medications such benzodiazepines alongside opioid analgesia.

13.4 Postoperative

13.4.1 Post-Anaesthetic Care Unit (PACU)/Recovery Room

Patients should be monitored in the PACU/recovery room postoperatively. Post-anaesthetic recovery should be in the sitting position to prevent further atelectasis. Supplemental oxygen should be administered to target preoperative SpO_2. Prior to discharge from PACU/recovery room, patients should be haemodynamic stable, alert and orientated, with acceptable pain scores and free from nausea or vomiting. Particular attention should be paid to the degree of oxygen requirement and the absence of apnoeic episodes prior to PACU/recovery room discharge.

13.4.2 Level of Postoperative Care

Patients should be managed at the level of care deemed most appropriate at pre-assessment. Resources should be available to escalate to a higher level of postoperative care should issues arise intraoperatively or postoperatively.

Risk scores can help establish the level of postoperative care required. The NCEPOD report found that high-risk patients admitted to critical care postoperatively had a mortality rate of 1.4% compared to 5% for those not admitted to critical care [1].

Patients with obesity should be considered for high dependency unit (HDU) postoperative care if they have been deemed as 'high risk' in perioperative risk assessment, have significant comorbidities, known OSA not established on CPAP, high risk for OSA on screening and not investigated/treated, known OSA or high risk on screening for OSA and likely to require high-dose opioids.

Particular care should be taken with patients with sleep-disordered breathing. The most suitable management and location of postoperative care for patients depending on OSA risk is suggested in Table 13.5. If patients with sleep-disordered breathing are suitable for ward-level care, oxygen should continue to be administered and SpO_2 monitored until SpO_2 has reached preoperative levels off oxygen.

Consideration for postoperative level of care should also take into account the complexity and duration of the surgical procedure. Short, minor surgical procedures that could be performed under regional anaesthesia carry less risk than prolonged complex surgeries under general anaesthesia where larger doses of perioperative opioids may be required.

13.4.3 Multimodal Analgesia

Postoperative pain management should be managed using a multimodal analgesia regime. Avoidance of opioids and sedatives is advised where possible to prevent airway or ventilation compromise. Patient-controlled analgesia (PCA) should be avoided where possible, particularly in patients with sleep-disordered breathing, due to the risk of respiratory depression. If a PCA is deemed necessary in patients with suspected or confirmed sleep-disordered breathing, they should be monitored in HDU postoperatively. If opioids are required, consideration should be given to continuous SpO_2 monitoring at ward level until mobilising postoperatively. If oral opioids are required, then immediate release forms are preferable. Slow-release opioids are not recommended for acute postoperative pain as they are associated with an increased risk of persistent use and respiratory depression [39].

13.4.4 Enhanced Recovery Programme

Patients should be enrolled in an enhanced recovery protocol for musculoskeletal surgery as for all other postoperative patients.

13.4.5 Venous Thromboembolism Prophylaxis

VTE prophylaxis should continue in the postoperative period. Postoperative management will be guided by preoperative risk assessment and type of surgical intervention. Early postoperative mobilisation should be encouraged. Most patients following musculoskeletal surgery should be encouraged to get out of the bed on the day of surgery. Thromboembolic deterrent stockings are generally continued until discharge. Pharmacological prophylaxis should be administered as soon as possible after surgery where the benefit is not outweighed by the risk of bleeding. Apixaban, aspirin, dabigatran, fondaparinux, rivaroxaban and low-molecular-weight heparin have all been used as VTE prophylaxis. Prophylactic anticoagulation dosing should take into account patients' weight. Pharmacotherapy is usually continued until the patients' mobility is no longer limited by the surgery. Doses may need to be held in order to facilitate epidural catheter removal [40]. If pharmacotherapy is contraindicated, consider intermittent pneumatic compression stockings.

13.5 Conclusion

Patients with obesity will present for musculoskeletal surgery at increasing frequency over the next number of years. Patients with obesity present specific challenges to anaesthesiologists in the perioperative period. With robust preoperative assessment, careful perioperative planning and awareness of the potential difficulties that may arise and how to mitigate these, anaesthesiologists can risk stratify and manage patients with obesity appropriately. Further research is needed in many areas, including the benefit or otherwise of preoperative weight loss and the dosing of drugs in patients with obesity.

References

1. Findlay G, Goodwin A, Protopapa K, Smith N, Mason M. Knowing the risk: a review of the peri-operative care of surgical patients. London: National Confidential Enquiry into Patient Outcome and Death (NCEPOD); 2011.
2. The Society for Obesity & Bariatric Anaesthesia. Anaesthesia for the obese patient. [Internet]. [cited 2023 Mar 13]. Available from: https://www.sobauk.co.uk/guidelines-1.
3. Weingarten TN, Flores AS, McKenzie JA, Nguyen LT, Robinson WB, Kinney TM, et al. Obstructive sleep apnoea and perioperative complications in bariatric patients. Br J Anaesth. 2011;106(1):131–9.
4. The Royal College of Surgeons of England Working Group on the Perioperative Care of the High-risk General Surgical Patient. The high-risk general surgical patient: raising the standard. London: The Royal College of Surgeons of England; 2018.
5. World Health Organization. Waist circumference and waist-hip ratio: report of a WHO expert consultation, Geneva, 8–11 December 2008. 2011. [cited 2023 Mar 13]. Available from: https://apps.who.int/iris/handle/10665/44583.
6. Committee on Economics. ASA physical status classification system [Internet]. American Society of Anaesthesiologists; 2020. Available from: https://www.asahq.org/standards-and-guidelines/asa-physical-status-classification-system.
7. Modig K, Erdefelt A, Mellner C, Cederholm T, Talbäck M, Hedström M. "Obesity paradox" holds true for patients with hip fracture: a registry-based cohort study. J Bone Joint Surg. 2019;101(10):888–95.
8. DeMaria EJ, Murr M, Byrne TK, Blackstone R, Grant JP, Budak A, et al. Validation of the obesity surgery mortality risk score in a multicenter study proves it stratifies mortality risk in patients undergoing gastric bypass for morbid obesity. Ann Surg. 2007;246(4):578–84.
9. Protopapa KL, Simpson JC, Smith NCE, Moonesinghe SR. Development and validation of the Surgical Outcome Risk Tool (SORT). Br J Surg. 2014;101(13):1774–83.

10. Bilimoria KY, Liu Y, Paruch JL, Zhou L, Kmiecik TE, Ko CY, et al. Development and evaluation of the universal ACS NSQIP surgical risk calculator: a decision aid and informed consent tool for patients and surgeons. J Am Coll Surg. 2013;217(5):833–42e3.
11. Sun Y, Liu B, Smith JK, Correia MLG, Jones DL, Zhu Z, et al. Association of preoperative body weight and weight loss with risk of death after bariatric surgery. JAMA Netw Open. 2020;3(5):e204803.
12. Cigrovski Berkovic M, Bilic-Curcic I, Mrzljak A, Canecki Varzic S, Cigrovski V. Prehabilitation of overweight and obese patients with dysglycemia awaiting bariatric surgery: predicting the success of obesity treatment. World J Diabetes. 2022;13(12):1096–105.
13. Purcell S, Hossain I, Evans B, Porter G, Richardson G, Ellsmere J. Morbid obesity and severe knee osteoarthritis: which should be treated first? J Gastrointest Surg. 2022;26(7):1388–93.
14. Wilding JPH, Batterham RL, Calanna S, Davies M, Van Gaal LF, Lingvay I, et al. Once-weekly semaglutide in adults with overweight or obesity. N Engl J Med. 2021;384(11):989–1002.
15. Bailey CR, Ahuja M, Bartholomew K, Bew S, Forbes L, Lipp A, et al. Guidelines for day-case surgery 2019: guidelines from the Association of Anaesthetists and the British Association of Day Surgery. Anaesthesia. 2019;74(6):778–92.
16. Joshi GP, Ankichetty SP, Gan TJ, Chung F. Society for ambulatory anesthesia consensus statement on preoperative selection of adult patients with obstructive sleep Apnea scheduled for ambulatory surgery. Anesth Analg. 2012;115(5):1060–8.
17. Brodsky JB. Positioning the morbidly obese patient for anesthesia. Obes Surg. 2002;12(6):751–8.
18. Douglass J, Fraser J, Andrzejowski J. Awake intubation and awake prone positioning of a morbidly obese patient for lumbar spine surgery. Anaesthesia. 2014;69(2):166–9.
19. Levy BJ, Tauberg BM, Holtzman AJ, Gruson KI. Reducing lateral femoral cutaneous nerve palsy in obese patients in the beach chair position: effect of a standardized positioning and padding protocol. J Am Acad Orthop Surg. 2019;27(12):437–43.
20. Gao D, Sun L, Wang N, Shi Y, Song J, Liu X, et al. Impact of 30° reserve Trendelenburg position on lung function in morbidly obese patients undergoing laparoscopic sleeve gastrectomy. Front Surg. 2022;9:792697.
21. Vaughan RW, Wise L. Intraoperative arterial oxygenation in obese patients. Ann Surg. 1976;184(1):35–42.
22. Members of the Working Party, Nightingale CE, Margarson MP, Shearer E, Redman JW, Lucas DN, et al. Peri-operative management of the obese surgical patient 2015: Association of Anaesthetists of Great Britain and Ireland Society for Obesity and Bariatric Anaesthesia. Anaesthesia. 2015;70(7):859–76.
23. Schumann R, Meidert AS, Bonney I, Koutentis C, Wesselink W, Kouz K, et al. Intraoperative blood pressure monitoring in obese patients. Anesthesiology. 2021;134(2):179–88.
24. National Guideline Centre (UK). Venous thromboembolism in over 16s: reducing the risk of hospital-acquired deep vein thrombosis or pulmonary embolism. London: National Institute for Health and Care Excellence; 2018.
25. Chin KJ, Perlas A, Chan V, Brown-Shreves D, Koshkin A, Vaishnav V. Ultrasound imaging facilitates spinal anesthesia in adults with difficult surface anatomic landmarks. Anesthesiology. 2011;115(1):94–101.
26. Parra MC, Loftus RW. Obesity and regional anesthesia. Int Anesthesiol Clin. 2013;51(3):90–112.
27. El Sherif FA, Othman AH, Abd El-Rahman AM, Taha O. Effect of adding intrathecal morphine to a multimodal analgesic regimen for postoperative pain management after laparoscopic bariatric surgery: a prospective, double-blind, randomized controlled trial. Br J Pain. 2016;10(4):209–16.
28. Schug SA, Scott PGM, David A, Halliwell AM, Richard MJ. Acute pain management: scientific evidence. 5th ed. Melbourne: Australian and New Zealand College of Anaesthetists, Faculty of Pain Medicine; 2020.
29. DeSousa KA. Intrathecal morphine for postoperative analgesia: current trends. World J Anesthesiol. 2014;3(3):191.

30. Cook T, Woodall N, Frerk C, editors. Major complications of airway management in the United Kingdom: report and findings: 4th National Audit Project of the Royal College of Anaesthetists and the Difficult Airway Society: NAP4. London: The Royal College of Anaesthetists; 2011.
31. Schutzer-Weissmann J, Wojcikiewicz T, Karmali A, Lukosiute A, Sun R, Kanji R, et al. Apnoeic oxygenation in morbid obesity: a randomised controlled trial comparing facemask and high-flow nasal oxygen delivery. Br J Anaesth. 2023;130(1):103–10.
32. Pandit JJ, Cook T, editors. Accidental awareness during general anaesthesia in the United Kingdom and Ireland: report and findings, September 2014; NAP5, 5th National Audit Project of the Royal College of Anaesthetists and the Association of Anaesthetists of Great Britain and Ireland. London: The Royal College of Anaesthetists; 2014.
33. Ingrande J, Lemmens HJM. Dose adjustment of anaesthetics in the morbidly obese. Br J Anaesth. 2010;105:i16–23.
34. O'Gara B, Talmor D. Perioperative lung protective ventilation. BMJ. 2018;362:k3030.
35. Wang C, Zhao N, Wang W, Guo L, Guo L, Chi C, et al. Intraoperative mechanical ventilation strategies for obese patients: a systematic review and network meta-analysis: mechanical ventilation for obese patient. Obes Rev. 2015;16(6):508–17.
36. Network ARDS, Brower RG, Matthay MA, Morris A, Schoenfeld D, Thompson BT, Wheeler A. Ventilation with lower tidal volumes as compared with traditional tidal volumes for acute lung injury and the acute respiratory distress syndrome. N Engl J Med. 2000;342(18):1301–8.
37. Gaszynski T, Szewczyk T, Gaszynski W. Randomized comparison of sugammadex and neostigmine for reversal of rocuronium-induced muscle relaxation in morbidly obese undergoing general anaesthesia. Br J Anaesth. 2012;108(2):236–9.
38. Stein PD, Beemath A, Olson RE, Obesity as a risk factor in venous thromboembolism. Am J Med. 2005;118(9):978–80.
39. Levy N, Mills P. Controlled-release opioids cause harm and should be avoided in management of postoperative pain in opioid naïve patients. Br J Anaesth. 2019;122(6):e86–90.
40. Kietaibl S, Ferrandis R, Godier A, Llau J, Lobo C, Macfarlane AJ, et al. Regional anaesthesia in patients on antithrombotic drugs: joint ESAIC/ESRA guidelines. Eur J Anaesthesiol. 2022;39(2):100–32.

Obesity and Musculoskeletal Imaging

14

Sarah K. Eustace, Stephen McLoughlin, Rosanne-Sara Lynham, and Stephen J. Eustace

Wealth and prosperity over the last decades have resulted in improved societal health and well-being. The average life expectancy in the developed world is now 73.5 years for a male and 79 years for a female (mean 76) versus expectancies of 53 years and 57 years, respectively, in some parts of the developing world. Unfortunately despite advantages for the majority, lifestyle changes and overavailability of poor food sources as part of prosperity have resulted in morbidity for a minority manifest by the development of excess corporal fat or obesity with associated healthcare problems: diabetes, hypertension, atherosclerosis, stroke, malignancies and musculoskeletal debility.

Such growth in the prevalence of obesity with associated effects on health is having a major impact on healthcare systems, medical and surgical across the world. This chapter, as part of a review of obesity and the musculoskeletal system, reviews the impact of obesity on medical imaging. Specifically, the chapter reviews technical issues presented to individual imaging modalities employed to image obese patients, the impact of obesity on interventional radiology and, finally, reviews the specific uses of imaging in obesity.

Radiology departments are now having to address issues not previously confronted such as what imaging modality would be most suitable to image the obese patient? How will the obese patient be transported to the radiology department? Will the patient's weight exceed limits for the imaging moving tabletop in a similar way to exceeding the weight limit for the surgical theatre tabletop? Will the patient be able to physically fit the imaging tunnel in computed tomography (CT) and magnetic resonance imaging (MRI) as the utilisation of imaging explodes and in parallel

S. K. Eustace · R.-S. Lynham (✉) · S. J. Eustace
National Orthopaedic Hospital Cappagh, Dublin, Ireland
e-mail: Saraheustace23@rcsi.ie; lynhamrs@tcd.ie

S. McLoughlin
University of Limerick, Limerick City, Ireland

J. M. O´Byrne et al. (eds.), *Musculoskeletal Disease and Obesity*,
https://doi.org/10.1007/978-3-031-63310-2_14

the prevalence of obesity in society grows, and these issues will be more frequently confronted? [1]. A 2006 study by Katz showed specific concerns from radiologists in being able to accurately read and report scans in obese patients due to sub-optimal scan results [2].

Obesity is defined as excessive body fat or a body mass index (BMI) of greater than 30 which considers height and weight. BMI can be useful for screening in obesity; however, without taking into account the different ethnicities, age groups and athletes, its efficacy has been questioned [3].

14.1 Practical/Physical Aspects of Obesity-Related Excess Weight and Body Diameter on Imaging

14.1.1 Patient Weight and Diameter

It is essential to document patient weight prior to imaging. Most imaging centres will have clearly documented table weight limits. Patients who exceed the standard weight limit for a given modality have the potential to damage equipment if it is used, leading to embarrassment for the patient and delaying imaging for other patients. The cost of damage to the technology will also not be covered by insurance, creating unnecessary costs for hospitals [4]. These table weight limits exist as increased weight on the table can limit the table mechanics.

An important factor to consider when choosing an imaging modality to use for a patient is the aperture diameter. The imaging modality may be able to accommodate a patient's weight but not diameter. The horizontal diameter is the widest section of the aperture in cross-sectional imaging. Vertical diameter should in theory be the same width as the horizontal diameter; however, they do not account for the table thickness entering the gantry or bore. The vertical dimension is usually approximately 15–18 cm smaller once the table thickness entering the gantry or bore has been excluded.

Patient girth is essential to ensure the patient safely fits in the machine. Patients' width is not usually measured prior to imaging; however, a solution that has been suggested is to use a hula hoop. If this is based on the dimensions of the largest diameter CT scanner, it will simply indicate whether the patients' girth exceeds the size of the machine [5].

It is now standard in many hospitals to have signs attached to imaging equipment detailing table weight and aperture limit [5]. These limits can be included in radiology software when ordering scans and alerts sent if the patients' weight exceeds the standard limits.

14.1.2 Physical Impact of Weight and Aperture Diameter: CT and MRI

Multidetector CT (MDCT) is the imaging technology of choice to image obese patients because it allows for the rapid acquisition of high-resolution images limiting the effects of claustrophobia and perspiration. Isotropic voxels facilitate multiplanar reconstructions. CT X-ray doses often need to be increased to minimise the impact of excess fat.

The CT standard gantry diameter is usually 70 cm with a standard table weight of 205 kg (450 lbs). With the increasing prevalence of obesity, there has been an increase in the availability of bariatric CT scanners which can measure up to 85 cm and allow for an increased weight of 308.44 kg (680 lbs).

The advantages of using MRI include lack of ionising radiation, better soft-tissue contrast than CT and hence the ability to better differentiate between fat, muscle and water. Slower image acquisition increases the impact of claustrophobia and perspiration.

MRI bore aperture is approximately 60 cm, and therefore, smaller than most CT scanners, and the table weight maximum is 159 kg (350lbs), significantly less than CT. Cylindrical bore MRI 1.5 T has a maximum aperture diameter of 70 cm (this has been a new development over recent years), whilst the vertical field MRI has a maximum aperture of 55 cm.

The development of 'open MRI units' has facilitated imaging of obese patients and can now accommodate patients with a girth greater than the MRI aperture diameter (approximately 70 cm). This is useful in imaging patients who exceed the 70 cm aperture diameter and weigh more than 205 kg; however, this leads to reduced quality images [6]. Most recently, Siemens has launched a new ultra-wide bore MRI with an aperture of 80 cm known as the Magnetom Free.Max, which is well suited for imaging obese patients and those who are claustrophobic.

14.1.3 Departmental Fluoroscopy: Theatre C Arm Imaging in Obesity

Fluoroscopy plays an important role in imaging patients' post-bariatric surgery, and in its mobile form, the C arm provides in-theatre real-time imaging.

Fluoroscopy typically rotates to create a relative aperture diameter of 45 cm; however, in centres where bariatric surgery is performed, they are required to have fluoroscopic equipment that can accommodate patients with wider girth and hence units with wider rotational circumferences are installed. New fluoroscopic equipment has made adjustments that can allow for an increased aperture diameter of 63 cm, This requires an over-couch tube and therefore comes with the risk of increased radiation dose [4].

The table weight for fluoroscopic equipment is the same as standard CT, 205 kg (450 lbs). Fluoroscopy differs from other imaging modalities in that weight limit, although contributory, is not necessarily the reason for not accommodating patients but more than the table width may not be able to accommodate the patient. The standard width for fluoroscopy is 45 cm which is often too narrow for obese patients [6].

C arm rotation can be limited by physical patient size. A wider rotational diameter overcomes this issue but increases scatter radiation to theatre staff with associated radiation safety implications.

14.1.4 General X-Ray and Obesity

Physical increase in patient size in obesity presents a significant technical issue when undertaking general X-ray.

The standard film cassette size is 14 × 17 inches. Often obese patients can exceed this limit and make imaging challenging. Knowledge of anatomical landmarks and the use of multiple cassettes to image quadrants of the body helps complete the imaging of body parts [6].

14.2 Impact of Obesity on the Quality of Diagnostic Images

Excess adipose tissue and thicker body parts require dose manipulation to provide high-quality images and maintain image contrast at the cost of increased patient radiation dose.

14.2.1 Radiography

To acquire high-quality images in obese patients requires manipulation of dose (KVp and Ma) and exposure time which is generally lengthened, resulting in an increased risk of subtle patient motion manifesting as artefact. The average setting for radiograph imaging is a kVp of approximately 90–95 and mAs of 2–2.5. Often these settings are not adequate to obtain high-quality images in obese patients and an increase in kVp and mAs is required to penetrate the soft tissue. This increases the risk of radiation-induced dose-dependent and non-dose-dependent effects to the patient.

Techniques to reduce radiation dose include increasing the tube voltage, positioning the patient with the thinnest layer of adipose tissue closest to the image receptor and the use of a moving grid to reduce the dose induced by scatter [7, 8].

14.2.2 Computed Tomography

Factors that reduce the quality of images in CT include increased exposure time, resulting in patient motion artefact, limited field of view, image cropping, increased noise and attenuation of the X-ray beams due to excessive soft tissue. Generally, if patients fit in the CT scanner good-quality images can be obtained.

CT Motion Artefact and Increased Noise: Inadequate beam penetration can result in increased noise. Some solutions to reducing noise include increasing the mAs and increasing the kVp to improve penetration. Both changes can decrease image contrast and increase the patient's radiation dose.

Motion artefact is less problematic in CT than in plain film radiograph; however, the increased time for photons to penetrate organs can cause solid organ margins to be less distinct [9].

CT Image Cropping: Once CT images have been obtained, a technologist may manually trim images to focus on a specific organ structure. In obese patients with increased subcutaneous fat, trimming these CT images may result in the loss of information about important pathology within the subcutaneous fat [10].

CT Limited Field of View/Beam Hardening: Most standard CT scanners with a gantry entry of 70 cm will have a field of view of 50–60 cm. Parts of patients' anatomy which extends beyond the field of view can result in beam hardening artefact and limit the evaluation of internal organs with imaging.

Increases in the gantry diameter (such as in special bariatric CT scanners) can lead to an extended field of view. Whilst this extended field of view can accommodate obese patients, it can also lead to distorted images [11].

The Benefits of Increased Adiposity in CT: Obesity may have some benefits in CT imaging of internal organs. Patients with an increased amount of retro/intraperitoneal fat have improved visualisation of internal organs as they are separated by fat; therefore, images are easier to interpret [12].

14.2.3 Magnetic Resonance Imaging

Excess corporal fat presents specific difficulties at MRI. Fat impedes radiofrequency penetration and hence tissue excitation which ultimately reduces acquired image signal. The field of view at MRI is limited to 55 cm, limiting complete imaging of specific body parts. Receiver coil placement is difficult, again reducing the image signal. To compensate for reduced image signal, multiple tissue excitations are employed which ultimately increases image acquisition time.

MRI Signal-to-Noise Ratio: MRI scanners with strong gradients cannot accommodate patients who are more than 60 cm in diameter or weigh more than 159 kg (350 lbs). In contrast, vertical open-field MRI scanners which can accommodate obese patients weighing more than 250 kg have weaker localising gradients and result in lower signal-to-noise ratios.

MRI Bore Length: Bore length is relevant in imaging obese patients with MRI. A long narrow bore (usually 170 cm) can cause discomfort and claustrophobia in obese patients. Shorter bore length magnets in MRI scanners may be preferable in obese patients so that their head/neck can be outside the bore.

MRI Limited Field of View: The standard field of view for a 1.5 T MRI ranges from 40 to 50 cm whilst the maximum field of view in a vertical open-field MRI is approximately 35–40 cm [13].

14.2.4 Ultrasound

The use of ultrasound in obese patients is extremely difficult primarily because fat reflects and attenuates sound, limiting tissue penetration and image creation.

In patients who weigh more than 250 lbs. and have fat predominantly in the subcutaneous tissues, sound penetration is markedly reduced, limiting visualisation of internal organs [4].

A number of solutions to these issues have been identified. Using a transducer with the lowest frequency, placing the transducer closest to the organ, pushing the transducer into the adipose tissue to decrease the penetrance depth, using a high-yield US machine/transducers and the use of harmonics are some examples [14].

14.2.5 Nuclear Medicine

Obesity creates a number of challenges to nuclear imaging. Radioisotope administration is based on patients' weight, meaning that obese patients may exceed the maximum dose allowed, and, therefore, as photons leave the body, they are attenuated by adipose tissue.

Obesity can also decrease the SNR, degrading the quality of images by the scatter of photons within the soft tissues. Increasing the maximum allowed dose of radioisotope and increasing the imaging time may improve image quality [12].

14.2.6 Mammography

Attenuation differences between fat, glandular tissue and tumours enhance the diagnostic value of mammograms.

However, when fat is excessive, issues such as limited tissue compression, the requirement for the increased dose to penetrate tissue and extended exposures with secondary motion all reduce image quality and diagnostic performance.

14.2.7 Interventional Radiology

Similar to other forms of imaging, patient weight and form present difficulties for the interventional radiologist.

The mechanical issues presented by excess subcutaneous and body fat present specific difficulties for percutaneous interventional procedures. Vessel cannulation can be difficult in thickened subcutaneous adipose tissues in which pulse detection for vessel localisation is obscured. Although ultrasound can be used for this purpose, it too is less valuable as images are distorted by sound attenuation and reflectivity induced by fat.

Excess subcutaneous fat limits the identification of surface landmarks which result in the need for image guidance to perform what are generally routine procedures such as knee injection.

Palpable landmarks for performing epidurals such as the sacral hiatus or shoulder injections are obscured and again can only be identified at fluoroscopy or even by using CT.

Radiation Dose: Obese patients usually require higher exposures to provide clear imaging guidance with associated biological risks.

Instrument Length and Imaging for Procedures: The standard length for most catheter wires is approximately 25 cm. Adipose tissue can create a greater than 25 cm distance between the skin and the target organ, making its use not possible. Optimised positioning of the patient with pillows to displace adipose tissue prior to the procedure and imaging beforehand to identify the shortest distance from skin to the target organ can obviate catheter length difficulties [3].

Sedation and Medications: Like radiation, increased doses of sedative medications are often required in obese patients, increasing the risk of respiratory depression. Worrying about respiratory depression or being unaware of the need for increased sedation disease obese patients may have procedures performed with inadequate sedation.

14.3 Specific Uses of Imaging in Obesity

14.3.1 Quantification of Total Body Fat

Recognising the limitations of simply weighing patients and measuring BMI, imaging is commonly employed to quantify total body fat content.

In this setting, DEXA scanning can be employed to create a planar image and separate bone from fat and fat from muscle by imaging at two different energy levels and creating an image based on the differential attenuation of two different low-energy X-ray beams.

CT scanning has been employed for the same purpose because CT images are acquired in slices, allowing 3D rather than planar assessment of total body fat and are therefore considerably more accurate than DEXA.

Employing whole-body MRI techniques, similar to CT but without the use of ionising radiation, MRI has been employed to quantify and follow changes in total body fat content.

14.3.2 Specific Diagnostic Imaging Appearances in Obesity

The distribution of body fat is dictated by male–female hormonal balance. In such a way, cross-sectional images acquired with CT and MRI show the characteristic distribution of body fat in men and women. Fat typically builds up within the abdomen in male obesity while it builds up in subcutaneous tissues in female obesity. In morbid obesity, the same distribution characteristics occur in men and women, although vast quantities of subcutaneous adipose tissue build up in both sexes. When it occurs, large fatty folds within the groin and axillary subcutaneous tissues, being immobile, can become engorged by disabled lymphatics and acquire a pseudo-tumour appearance (Figs. 14.1 and 14.2).

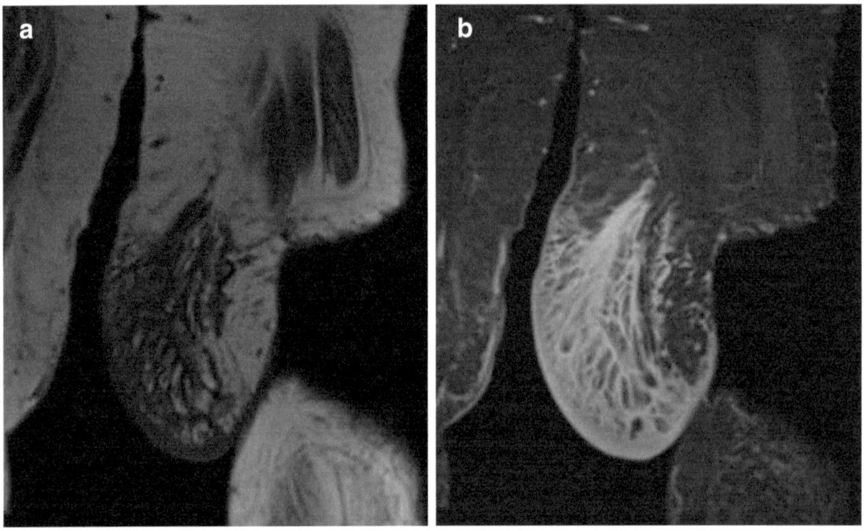

Fig. 14.1 Pseudosarcoma of the morbidly obese: massive localised lymphoedema. (**a**) T1 weighted image of groin fold showing tumour-like proliferation of fat with secondary lymphoedema simulating sarcoma. (**b**) T2 weighted image of the same patient showing acquired lymphoedema

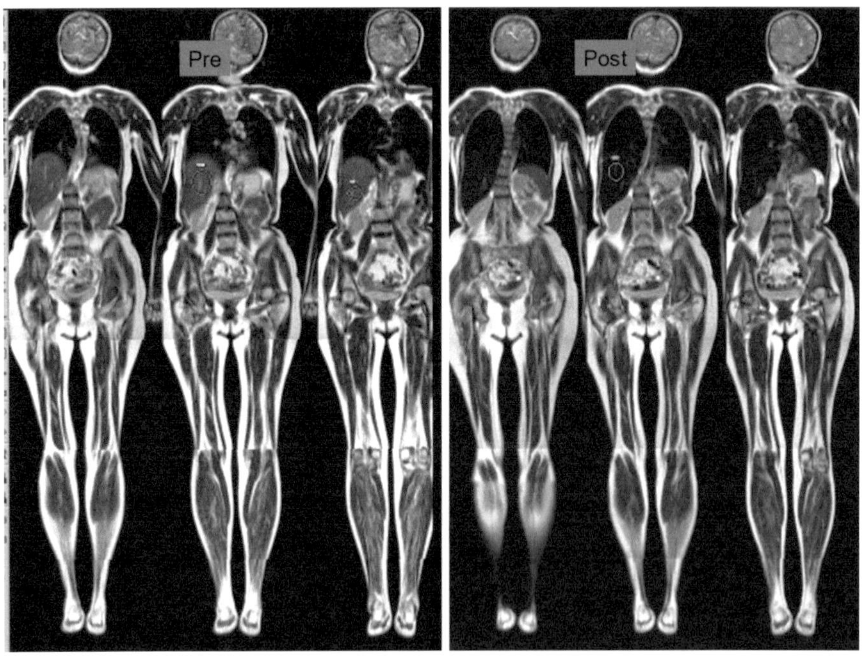

Fig. 14.2 T1 weighted whole-body MRI employed to quantify total body fat. Fat identified as hyperintense on T1 weighted imaging

In anorexia nervosa where subcutaneous tissues have become completely catabolised, patients start to catabolise fat within the marrow space, fat becoming replaced by fluid in a process termed liquefactive necrosis (Fig. 14.3).

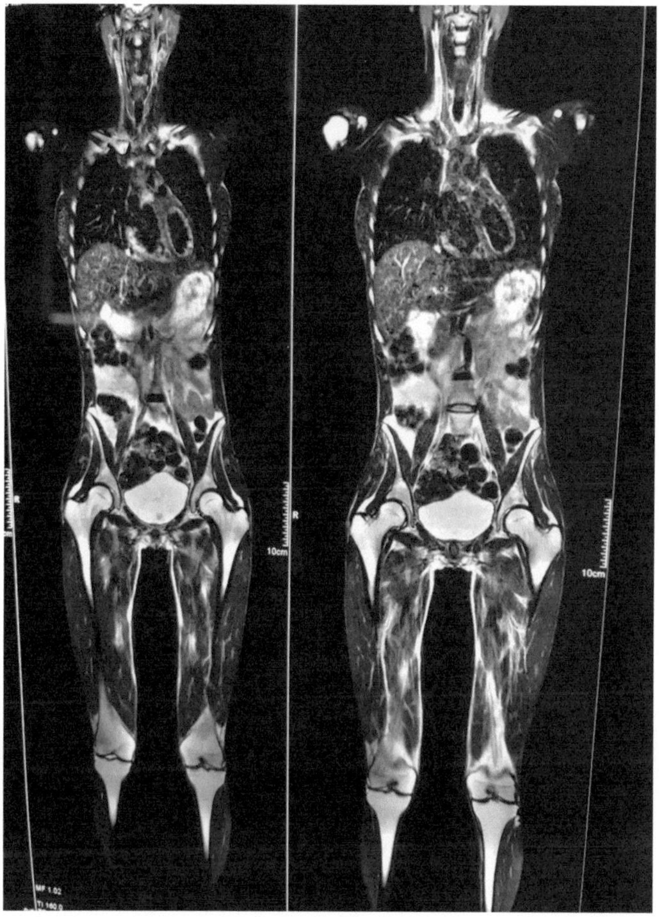

Fig. 14.3 Liquefactive necrosis in a severe anorexic characterised by fluid within the marrow space on this whole-body fat-suppressed STIR image

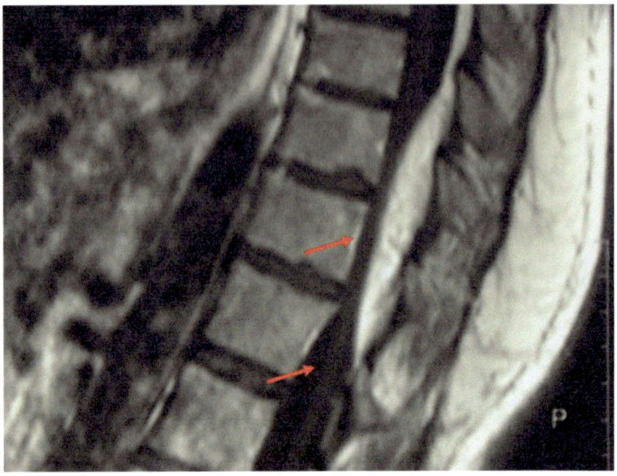

Fig. 14.4 Epidural fat proliferation termed epidural lipomatosis presenting with signs of thecal sac compression

In contrast, excess fat can become identified in usual areas such as the epidural space and lead to thecal sac compression termed epidural lipomatosis (Fig. 14.4).

References

1. Uppot RN. Impact of obesity on radiology. Radiol Clin North Am. 2007;45(2):231–46.
2. Katz A. Obesity impedes medical imaging. New Haven Register. 2006.
3. Widhalm K, Schönegger K, Huemer C, Auterith A. Does the BMI reflect body fat in obese children and adolescents? A study using the TOBEC method. Int J Obes Relat Metab Disord. 2001;25(2):279–85.
4. Uppot RN, Sahani DV, Hahn PF, Gervais D, Mueller PR. Impact of obesity on medical imaging and image-guided intervention. AJR Am J Roentgenol. 2007;188:433–40.
5. Ginde AA, Foianini A, Renner DM, Valley M, Camargo CA. The challenge of CT and MRI imaging of obese individuals who present to the emergency department: a national survey. Obesity. 2008;16:2549–51.
6. Carucci LR. Imaging obese patients: problems and solutions. Abdom Imaging. 2013;38:630–46.
7. Mileto A, Samei E, Huo D, Rill L. Hallway conversations in physics. AJR Am J Roentgenol. 2017;208:W56–7.
8. Yanch JC, Behrman RH, Hendricks MJ, McCall JH. Increased radiation dose to overweight and obese patients from radiographic examinations. Radiology. 2009;252:128–39.
9. Beeksma B, Truant D, Holloway L, Arumugam S. An assessment of image distortion and CT number accuracy within a wide-bore CT extended field of view. Australas Phys Eng Sci Med. 2015;38:255–61.
10. Fursevich DM, LiMarzi GM, O'Dell MC, Hernandez MA, Sensakovic WF. Bariatric CT imaging: challenges and solutions. Radiographics. 2016;36:1076–86.
11. Uppot RN. Technical challenges of imaging & image-guided interventions in obese patients. Br J Radiol. 2018;91:20170931.

12. Uppot R, Sheehan A, Seethamraju R. Obesity and MR imaging. AJR. 2007;188:433–40.
13. Sabati M, Lauzon ML, Mahallati H, Frayne R. Interactive continuously moving table (iCMT) large field-of-view real-time MRI. Magn Reson Med. 2006;55:1202–9.
14. Shapiro RS, Wagreich J, Parsons RB, Stancato-Pasik A, Yeh HC, Lao R. Tissue harmonic imaging sonography: evaluation of image quality compared with conventional sonography. AJR Am J Roentgenol. 1998;171:1203–6.

Prehabilitation and Rehabilitation Issues 15

Fred Kenny, Ailbhe Rogan, and Colin Dunlevy

15.1 Introduction

Obesity is a complex chronic disease, characterised by dysfunctional or excess body fat (adiposity) that impairs health [1]. This disease is associated with a lower quality of life and a higher prevalence of concomitant disease with poorer health outcomes compared to the population without obesity [2].

The reasons for this reduction in health outcomes and quality of life are multifactorial and often interdependent. An example of this multidirectional relationship that is central to this chapter is that of the relationship between chronic musculoskeletal (MSk) pain, adaptive behaviour, physical function and health outcome.

The International Association for the Study of Pain (IASP) (2020) defines pain as 'an unpleasant sensory and emotional experience associated with, or resembling that associated with, actual or potential tissue damage'; the consensus statement further explains that pain has adverse effects on physical function and psychosocial well-being.

A person experiencing pain due to osteoarthritis (OA) or other MSk disease typically behaves in a way that avoids painful aggravating stimuli, which often results in a lowering of the person's habitual movement and total daily physical activity (PA) [3]. If the pain is chronic, a 'fear avoidance' behaviour may become established. This chronic lowering of PA and avoidance of routine physical demands may result in a deterioration of a person's aerobic capacity and muscle atrophy and

F. Kenny (✉)
National Orthopaedic Hospital Cappagh, Dublin, Ireland

A. Rogan
Dublin City University, Dublin, Ireland

C. Dunlevy
Centre for Obesity Management, St. Columcille's Hospital, Dublin, Ireland
e-mail: Colin.Dunlevy@hse.ie

J. M. O´Byrne et al. (eds.), *Musculoskeletal Disease and Obesity*,
https://doi.org/10.1007/978-3-031-63310-2_15

function. These changes are associated with an adverse influence on morbidity and mortality [9] and worsening MSk disease [10].

Pain is highly prevalent in the population of people living with obesity (PLwO), with one Irish study reporting significant pain in 91% of patients [4]. It has also been shown that PLwO and pain have poorer physical function compared to those without pain [7]. For those seeking treatment for their obesity, the presence of pain is associated with lower changes to body weight [5, 6]. This finding of a reduced capacity to influence body weight helps us understand the complexity of obesity and illustrates the bidirectional relationship between pain and obesity.

15.2 Treating Obesity, Pain and Musculoskeletal Disease

Despite the simplistic motto of 'eat less, move more', research has shown us that this approach is not curative for obesity [8] and has only a modest influence on body weight reduction of about 4 kg [11]. That is not to say that a patient's relationship with food, physical activity and other habitual behaviours does not influence the disease of obesity. These remain as central tenants for a wide variety of chronic diseases, including obesity care. However, like other chronic diseases, such as hypertension, we recommend optimising physical activity and dietary habits in order to improve outcomes rather than use them to evoke disease remission [12].

For the general population, higher physical activity (PA) levels and lower sedentary (sitting) time are associated with improved cardiovascular health outcomes, such as blood pressure, low-density lipoprotein-cholesterol (LDL-C), triglycerides, glucose, high-density lipoprotein-cholesterol (HDL-C) levels, visceral fat and a lower incidence of chronic disease [e.g. type 2 diabetes mellitus (T2DM), cardiovascular disease (CVD), certain types of cancer] [18, 19].

15.3 Physical Activity and Obesity Care

PLwO face stigmatising attitudes when seeking healthcare [13, 14]. The basis for these negative experiences may be based in part on the misplaced belief by some healthcare professionals (HCPs) that the patient has not taken responsibility for their health or appropriate action to manage their body weight through burning sufficient calories. This intuitive understanding of calorie burning and its influence on energy balance is known as the 'additive model' of energy expenditure. The premise is that a defined bout of PA is associated with a defined number of calories used. These calories are provided by the body's internal store of adiposity. Therefore, if a patient 'moves more' they will use up the excess adiposity and will lose weight. It seems this rudimentary understanding of body weight regulation persists despite many studies showing that this is a false premise as it is now understood that the body has many adaptive processes to prevent weight loss that is brought about by increasing PA and energy demands. A recent study by Careau et al. (2021) [15] used the doubly labelled water technique, which is the gold standard technique to assess human energy expenditure in real-world settings, to examine daily energy expenditure in 1754 Europeans. In consensus with previous works, this study dismissed the 'additive model' of energy expenditure and instead endorsed the 'compensation model'. This model illustrates how our physiology has homeostatic mechanisms to regulate the amount of energy that it will use over a typical day. Additionally, they state that PLwO demonstrate higher levels of compensation within its energy regulation systems. Therefore, after a period of weight loss this physiological compensation within our bodies creates what is known as the 'energy gap' and may serve to increase the drive for body weight to return back to baseline.

While maintaining an active lifestyle has been shown to be helpful in long-term weight maintenance [16], one of the most important functions of promoting routine PA for this population is in the maintenance of physical function, cardiovascular health and mental health all of which may be compromised by the disease of obesity [16, 17].

Additionally in the context of pain management, exercise programmes in combination with dietary strategies have been shown to have a positive effect on pain outcome for PLwO, whereas dietary strategies by themselves had no effect on pain [17]. Pozzobon et al. (2018) also linked higher PAL with improved outcomes in pain and function following orthopaedic procedures [40].

In summary, PA counselling is very important for PLwO to help manage both OA and pain. It has been shown to improve physical function and pain score in addition to lowering morbidity and mortality. However, patient consultations should avoid discussing PA as a means to burn off excess adipose tissue as the disease of obesity is characterised by this complex physiological issue and is not resolved by the reductive notion of simply moving more.

15.4 Prehabilitation and Preparation for Surgery

As with all patient populations undergoing orthopaedic surgery, a planned pathway is fundamental to optimise outcomes. When preparing for surgery in addition to routine blood tests and investigations such as ECG or echo, a prehabilitation programme is often initiated. A prehabilitation programme can consist of education, exercise to increase both muscle function and cardiovascular health and may also include psychological and nutritional counselling. The rationale for a prehabilitation programme is that an individual may maintain a higher level of functional ability and rebound more rapidly post surgery if they are adequately prepared using a standard programme [25, 33].

There is evidence that prehabilitation can reduce admission to rehabilitation centres postoperatively [21, 22]. However, a lower certainty of evidence that prehabilitation can improve many other postoperative outcomes in the general population [20, 21]. One systematic review suggests that there was no significant benefit in the functional, quality of life or pain outcomes after knee and hip arthroplasty for those in the general population who participated in a prehabilitation programme [22].

However, prehabilitation has been suggested as important for specific patient subgroups, including PLwO [25]. It has been reported that orthopaedic procedures hold increased risk for some of these populations [25, 40]. For PLwO it has research shows that there are higher rates of site infection, surgical revision, blood loss, venous thromboembolism, length of stay and overall costs in joint arthroplasty [30, 40]. The increased risk rates vary from minimal to substantial depending on the profile of the PLwO and their concomitant disease status [26, 29].

Diseases such as type 2 diabetes, cardiovascular disease, hypertension and obstructive sleep apnoea seem to have a higher risk loading than obesity alone. For example, according to the American College of Surgeons risk calculator, a functionally independent 64-year-old woman with a BMI of 57 kg/m^2 undergoing a total knee arthroplasty (TKA) who has a history of mild system disease has only a 0.5% increased risk of surgical site infection, and no other increased risks of postoperative complications compared to the general population. However, if the same patient has severe systemic disease, is partially dependent and has both type 2 diabetes and hypertension, their risks across most post-surgical complications increase from no increase for mortality [27, 28] to an additional 8% increase in the risk of requiring convalescence.

15.5 Pre-Surgery Consolations

As previously discussed, obesity as a singular diagnosis provides limited predictors regarding the risks associated with orthopaedic procedures and should be considered with a more in-depth medical history. Similarly, the type of orthopaedic procedure will have a substantial bearing on both the surgical risk and considerations for the rehabilitation process. For example, obesity has not been shown as a reliable predictor of outcomes for upper limb surgeries and does not have special considerations attached [43].

Given these variations in risk, blanket statements about the increased risk for orthopaedic surgery for those PLwO should be avoided in favour of a tailored approach given the individual patients' wider health status. The tone of these discussions should reflect the nature of obesity as a chronic disease. The HCP should avoid stigmatising language as this has been shown to influence patient participation, is associated with poorer health and obesity outcomes and is viewed as counterproductive [14].

The focus of the consultation should be on health gain, risk management and setting expectations rather than weight loss. Weight loss is not something that a patient can directly control. In fact, the patient may have already lost a clinically significant amount of weight and have attained a good level of physical fitness prior to their orthopaedic consultation.

Furthermore, while modest weight loss can improve important health markers, it has also been shown to have the potential to have a negative effect on surgical outcomes. This may be due to its association with rebound weight gain postoperatively and the possibility that there was excessive muscle loss during the weight reduction phase [31, 32].

If the preoperative consultation acknowledges the individual's weight management history to that point, an informed conversation with directed and realistic prehabilitation goals can be set. This will be more beneficial than a conversation based on unrealistic weight-related goals. Typical worthwhile goals may include strategies regarding localised strengthening work, general aerobic fitness, nutritional counselling, a medication review and arranging for other screenings such as for obstructive sleep apnoea or a dental review.

Obesity Canada has provided a worthwhile evidence-based framework to guide HCPs towards helpful conversation in obesity care. This framework is called 'the 5 A's'. It suggests the HCP should follow simple headings when they have a healthcare consultation with PLwO. These headings are assess, advise, agree, assist and arrange. Further details on this approach are readily available [45].

15.6 Equipment

As a basic requirement, equipment and procedures should be suitable for higher body weights. With the high prevalence of obesity in the health-seeking population, equipment such as chairs, blood pressure cuffs, mobility aids, beds, commodes, hoists and trollies should have an appropriate safe working load of no less than 250 kg. There should also be contingency plans for even higher body weights that may present in emergency situations. Further information regarding appropriate clinical equipment can be found via the Association for the Study of Obesity Ireland (ASOI) [44].

15.7 Post-Surgery Rehabilitation

The goal of a rehabilitation programme following orthopaedic surgery will be to restore physical function to an optimal level using targeted strengthening, range of movement and functional exercises in addition to other adaptive strategies, including the use of aids and appliances. Rehabilitation has been proven to give significant improvement in functional outcomes following orthopaedic surgery. This has been shown to be true for the general population and PLwO [23]. There are strong parallels between the multidisciplinary team (MDT) management of orthopaedic rehabilitation and a specialist obesity care service. Both interventions will provide a supportive environment with tailored and achievable rehabilitation goals. HCPs will provide problem-solving support and a structured programme for these complex healthcare issues.

Although there may be some special consideration when rehabilitating PLwO, for example, an individual's improvements may be at a slower rate [23], require equipment with appropriate safe working loads and may have some financial implications regarding the total cost of treatment [34, 35]. These issues will vary depending on the type of surgery and the wider health profile of the patient.

There are variations in reported outcomes for different types of orthopaedic surgery for PLwO. Understanding these may help guide expectations and help rehabilitation to be directed.

TKAs have shown inferior outcomes in only short-term metrics for PLwO with longer term functional outcomes being similar to the general population [36, 38]. Whereas other studies found no significant difference in the groups after the same surgeries [37]. Yet, another study found that postoperative improvement in joint-specific outcomes was larger in PLwO compared to the general population [39]. These findings suggest that once the patient manages to avoid surgical-site complications and there is suitable equipment available with the appropriate safe working loads, there are no specific rehabilitation concerns for TKA with PLwO.

For total hip arthroplasty (THA), some authors have reported that while there is an equal gain in post-surgery outcomes, PLwO are less likely to attain the same functional level when compared to the general population [35, 40]. One longer term study found that at 10 years there were no significant differences in hip pain or function between the PLwO and those without obesity. However, PLwO had poorer walking capacity, were more likely to use walking aids and were less satisfied with the outcome [24]. This may indicate that the rehabilitation process for THA should address these expectations and highlight the need for long-term maintenance of walking ability and continued strength work.

In orthopaedic trauma patients, obesity adds to the risk and complexity of surgery. Evidence based on BMI cutoffs has shown that PLwO are at higher risk for nerve injuries, intraoperative complications, increased blood loss, increased operative times and non-union [41, 42, 43]. It is reasonable to say that these will have an effect on the patient's rehabilitation and may influence long-term outcomes.

Careful preoperative planning and specialised rehabilitation can give PLwO the best opportunity for a good outcome [43]. As with the previous examples, risk management, functional and pain outcomes should be based on a global view of the patient's medical history and baseline function rather than merely based on BMI cutoffs.

References

1. Courtney A, Harrington JM, Murrin C. Adult obesity clinical practice guideline adaptation (ASOI version 1, 2022). Chapter adapted from: Twells LK, Janssen I, Kuk JL. Available from: https://asoi.info/guidelines/epidemiology/. Accessed Feb 2023.
2. Gupta S, Richard L, Forsythe A. The humanistic and economic burden associated with increasing body mass index in the EU5. Diabetes Metab Syndr Obes. 2015;8:327–38.
3. Alzahrani H, Mackey M, Stamatakis E, Zadro JR, Shirley D. The association between physical activity and low back pain: a systematic review and meta-analysis of observational studies. Sci Rep. 2019;9(1):1–10.
4. MacLellan GA, Dunlevy C, O'Malley E, Blake C, Breen C, Gaynor K, et al. Musculoskeletal pain profile of obese individuals attending a multidisciplinary weight management service. Pain. 2017;158(7):1342–53.

5. Masheb RM, Lutes LD, Kim HM, Holleman RG, Goodrich DE, Janney CA, et al. Weight loss outcomes in patients with pain. Obesity (Silver Spring). 2015;23(9):1778–84. https://doi.org/10.1002/oby.21160.
6. Ryan CG, Vijayaraman A, Denny V, Ogier A, Ells L, Wellburn S, et al. The association between baseline persistent pain and weight change in patients attending a specialist weight management service. PLoS One. 2017;12(6):e0179227. https://doi.org/10.1371/journal.pone.0179227.
7. Dunlevy C, MacLellan GA, O'Malley E, Blake C, Breen C, Gaynor K, et al. Does changing weight change pain? Retrospective data analysis from a national multidisciplinary weight management service. Eur J Pain. 2019;23(8):1403–15.
8. Breen C, O'Connell J, Geoghegan J, O'Shea D, Birney S, Tully L, et al. Obesity in adults: A 2022 adapted clinical practice guideline for Ireland. Obes Facts. 2022;15(6):736–52.
9. Torrance N, Elliott AM, Lee AJ, Smith BH. Severe chronic pain is associated with increased 10 year mortality. A cohort record linkage study. Eur J Pain. 2010;14:380–6.
10. Vlietstra L, Stebbings S, Meredith-Jones K, Abbott JH, Treharne GJ, Waters DL. Sarcopenia in osteoarthritis and rheumatoid arthritis: the association with self-reported fatigue, physical function and obesity. PLoS One. 2019;14(6):e0217462.
11. Boulé NG, Prud'homme D. Canadian adult obesity clinical practice guidelines: physical activity in obesity management. Available from: https://obesitycanada.ca/guidelines/physicalactivity. Accessed 7 Mar 2023.
12. Pescatello LS, Buchner DM, Jakicic JM, Powell KE, Kraus WE, Bloodgood B, et al. Physical activity to prevent and treat hypertension: a systematic review. Med Sci Sports Exerc. 2019;51(6):1314–23.
13. O'Donoghue G, Cunningham C, King M, O'Keefe C, Rofaeil A, McMahon S. A qualitative exploration of obesity bias and stigma in Irish healthcare; the patients' voice. PLoS One. 2021;16(11):e0260075.
14. Tomiyama AJ. Stress and obesity. Annu Rev Psychol. 2019;70:703–18.
15. Careau V, Halsey LG, Pontzer H, Ainslie PN, Andersen LF, Anderson LJ, et al. Energy compensation and adiposity in humans. Curr Biol. 2021;31(20):4659–66.e2.
16. Dunlevy C, Gregg E, Woods C, O'Malley G. SOI adult obesity clinical practice guideline adaptation (ASOI version 1, 2022). Chapter adapted from: Boulé NG, Prud'homme D. Available from: https://asoi.info/guidelines/physicalactivity/. Accessed 15 Mar 2023.
17. Hall M, Castelein B, Wittoek R, Calders P, Van Ginckel A. Diet-induced weight loss alone or combined with exercise in overweight or obese people with knee osteoarthritis: a systematic review and meta-analysis. Semin Arthritis Rheum. 2019;48(5):765–77.
18. Warburton DE, Nicol CW, Bredin SS. Health benefits of physical activity: the evidence. CMAJ. 2006;174(6):801–9.
19. de Rezende LF, Rodrigues Lopes M, Rey-Lopez JP, Matsudo VK, Luiz OC. Sedentary behavior and health outcomes: an overview of systematic reviews. PLoS One. 2014;9(8):e105620.
20. Briguglio M, Wahhainwright TW. Nutritional and physical prehabilitation in elective orthopedic surgery: rationale and proposal for implementation. Ther Clin Risk Manag. 2022;18:21–30. https://doi.org/10.2147/tcrm.s341953.
21. McIsaac DI, Gill M, Boland L, Hutton B, Branje K, Shaw J, Grudzinski AL, Barone N, Gillis C, Akhtar S, Atkins M, Aucoin S, Auer R, Basualdo-Hammond C, Beaule P, Brindle M, Bittner H, Bryson G, Carli F, Eskander A, Fata P, Fergusson D, Fiore J, Forster A, Gillam M, Gramlich L, Holroyd-Leduc J, Jackson T, Jacobsohn E, Khadaroo R, Lalu M, Love C, Martel G, McCartney C, McKeen D, Meliambro A, Moloo H, Moore R, Muscedere J, Nantel J, Poitras S, Scheede-Bergdahl C, Taljaard M, Wallace T, Wijeysundera D. Prehabilitation in adult patients undergoing surgery: an umbrella review of systematic reviews. Br J Anaesth. 2022;128(2):244–57. https://doi.org/10.1016/j.bja.2021.11.014.
22. Cabilan CJ, Hines S, Munday J. The effectiveness of prehabilitation or preoperative exercise for surgical patients: a systematic review. JBI Database Syst Rev Implement Rep. 2015;13(1):146–87. https://doi.org/10.11124/jbisrir-2015-1885.

23. Vincent HK, Seay AN, Vincent KR, Atchison JW, Sadasivan K. Effects of obesity on rehabilitation outcomes after orthopedic trauma. Am J Phys Med Amp Rehabil. 2012;91(12):1051–9. https://doi.org/10.1097/phm.0b013e31825f1b19.
24. Baillot A, Chenail S, Barros Polita N, Simoneau M, Libourel M, Nazon E, et al. Physical activity motives, barriers, and preferences in people with obesity: a systematic review. PLoS One. 2021;16(6):e0253114. https://doi.org/10.1371/journal.pone.0253114.
25. Wall C, de Steiger R. Pre-operative optimisation for hip and knee arthroplasty: minimise risk and maximise recovery. Aust J Gen Pract. 2020;49(11):710–4. https://doi.org/10.31128/ajgp-05-20-5436.
26. Carreira D, Robison JW, Robison S, Fitch A. Obesity treatment in orthopaedic surgery. J Am Acad Orthop Surg. 2022;30(24):e1563–70. https://doi.org/10.5435/jaaos-d-21-01083.
27. Dowsey MM, Choong PF, Paxton EW, Spelman T, Namba RS, Inacio MC. Body mass index is associated with all-cause mortality after THA and TKA. Clin Orthop Relat Res. 2018;476(6):1139–48. https://doi.org/10.1007/s11999.0000000000000108.
28. Evans JT, Mouchti S, Blom AW, Wilkinson JM, Whitehouse MR, Beswick A, et al. Obesity and revision surgery, mortality, and patient-reported outcomes after primary knee replacement surgery in the National Joint Registry: A UK cohort study. PLoS Med. 2021;18(7):e1003704. https://doi.org/10.1371/journal.pmed.1003704.
29. Memtsoudis SG, Besculides MC, Gaber L, Liu S, Valle GDA. Risk factors for pulmonary embolism after hip and knee arthroplasty: a population-based study. Int Orthop. 2008;33(6):1739–45. https://doi.org/10.1007/s00264-008-0659-z.
30. McElroy M, Pivec R, Issa K, Harwin S, Mont M. The effects of obesity and morbid obesity on outcomes in TKA. J Knee Surg. 2013;26(02):083–8. https://doi.org/10.1055/s-0033-1341407.
31. Wu M, Cochrane NH, Kim B, Belay ES, O'Donnell J, Ryan SP, et al. Patterns and predictors of weight change before and after total hip arthroplasty in class 2 and 3 obese patients. J Arthroplast. 2022;37(5):880–7. https://doi.org/10.1016/j.arth.2022.01.009.
32. Kim BI, Cochrane NH, O'Donnell JA, Wu M, Wellman SS, Ryan S, et al. Preoperative weight loss and postoperative weight gain independently increase risk for revision after primary total knee arthroplasty. J Arthroplast. 2022;37(4):674–82. https://doi.org/10.1016/j.arth.2021.12.003.
33. Ditmyer MM, Topp R, Pifer M. Prehabilitation in preparation for orthopaedic surgery. Orthop Nurs. 2002;21(5):43–54. https://doi.org/10.1097/00006416-200209000-00008.
34. Vincent HK, Vincent KR. Obesity and inpatient rehabilitation outcomes following knee arthroplasty: a multicenter study. Obesity. 2008;16(1):130–6. https://doi.org/10.1038/oby.2007.10.
35. Vincent HK, Weng JP, Vincent KR. Effect of obesity on inpatient rehabilitation outcomes after total hip arthroplasty. Obesity. 2007;15(2):522–30. https://doi.org/10.1038/oby.2007.551.
36. Baum G, Jacobs H, Lazovic D, Maus U, Hoffmann F, Seeber GH. The influence of obesity on functional outcomes and patient satisfaction 8 weeks after total knee arthroplasty: results of the prospective FInGK study. BMC Musculoskelet Disord. 2022;23(1):949. https://doi.org/10.1186/s12891-022-05874-w.
37. Baghbani-Naghadehi F, Armijo-Olivo S, Prado CM, Gramlich L, Woodhouse LJ. Does obesity affect patient-reported outcomes following total knee arthroplasty? BMC Musculoskelet Disord. 2022;23(1):55. https://doi.org/10.1186/s12891-022-04997-4.
38. Giesinger JM, Loth FL, MacDonald DJ, Giesinger K, Patton JT, Simpson AH, et al. Patient-reported outcome metrics following total knee arthroplasty are influenced differently by patients' body mass index. Knee Surg Sports Traumatol Arthrosc. 2018;26(11):3257–64. https://doi.org/10.1007/s00167-018-4853-2.
39. Giesinger K, Giesinger J, Hamilton D, Rechsteiner J, Ladurner A. Higher body mass index is associated with larger postoperative improvement in patient-reported outcomes following total knee arthroplasty. BMC Musculoskelet Disord. 2021;22(1):635. https://doi.org/10.1186/s12891-021-04512-1.
40. Pozzobon D, Ferreira PH, Blyth FM, Machado GC, Ferreira ML. Can obesity and physical activity predict outcomes of elective knee or hip surgery due to osteoarthritis? A

meta-analysis of cohort studies. BMJ Open. 2018;8(2):e017689. https://doi.org/10.1136/bmjopen-2017-017689.
41. Lazar MA, Plocher EK, Egol KA. Obesity and its relationship with pelvic and lower-extremity orthopedic trauma. Am J Orthop (Belle Mead NJ). 2010;39(4):175–82.
42. Purcell KF, Bergin PF, Spitler CA, Graves ML, Russell GV. Management of pelvic and acetabular fractures in the obese patient. Orthop Clin North Am. 2018;49(3):317–24. https://doi.org/10.1016/j.ocl.2018.02.005.
43. Spitler CA, Hulick RM, Graves ML, Russell GV, Bergin PF. Obesity in the polytrauma patient. Orthop Clin N Am. 2018;49(3):307–15.
44. Duggan D, Kearney C, Hynes M, Manning S, O'Malley E. ASOI adult obesity clinical practice guideline adaptation (ASOI version 1, 2022). Chapter adapted from: Rueda-Clausen C, Poddar M, Lear S, Poirier P, Sharma A. Available from: https://asoi.info/guidelines/assessment/. Accessed 16 Mar 2023.
45. https://obesitycanada.ca/resources/5as/. Accessed 16 Mar 2023.

MIX
Papier aus verantwortungsvollen Quellen
Paper from responsible sources
FSC® C105338
FSC
www.fsc.org

If you have any concerns about our products,
you can contact us on
ProductSafety@springernature.com

In case Publisher is established outside the EU,
the EU authorized representative is:
Springer Nature Customer Service Center GmbH
Europaplatz 3, 69115 Heidelberg, Germany

Printed by Libri Plureos GmbH
in Hamburg, Germany